Sirtfood Diet

The Ultimate Guide to Quickly Lose Weight, Burn Stubborn Fat, and Activate the Skinny Gene with a 21-Day Meal Plan, Including a Cookbook with Delicious Recipes

Text Copyright © [Thomas Slow]

All rights reserved. No part of this guide may be reproduced in any form without permission in writing from the publisher except in the case of brief quotations embodied in critical articles or reviews.

Legal & Disclaimer

The information contained in this book and its contents is not designed to replace or take the place of any form of medical or professional advice; and is not meant to replace the need for independent medical, financial, legal or other professional advice or services, as may be required. The content and information in this book has been provided for educational and entertainment purposes only.

The content and information contained in this book has been compiled from sources deemed reliable, and it is accurate to the best of the Author's knowledge, information and belief. However, the Author cannot guarantee its accuracy and validity and cannot be held liable for any errors and/or omissions. Further, changes are periodically made to this book as and when needed. Where appropriate and/or necessary, you must consult a professional (including but not limited to your doctor, attorney, financial advisor or such other professional advisor) before using any of the suggested remedies, techniques, or information in this book.

Upon using the contents and information contained in this book, you agree to hold harmless the Author from and against any damages, costs, and expenses, including any legal fees potentially resulting from the application of any of the information provided by this book. This disclaimer applies to any loss, damages or injury caused by the use and application, whether directly or indirectly, of any advice or information presented, whether for breach of contract, tort, negligence, personal injury, criminal intent, or under any other cause of action.

You agree to accept all risks of using the information presented inside this book.

You agree that by continuing to read this book, where appropriate and/or necessary, you shall consult a professional (including but not limited to your doctor, attorney, or financial advisor or such other advisor as needed) before using any of the suggested remedies, techniques, or information in this book.

Table of Contents

WHAT IS THE SIRTFOOD DIET? 9
IS IT REALLY EFFECTIVE? 13
HOW TO ADHERE TO THE SIRTFOOD DIET 18
SIRTFOOD DIET -- PHASE ONE 26
SIRTFOOD DIET -- PHASE TWO 32
GETTING STARTED: GROCERY LIST 43
BREAKFAST RECIPES 53
LUNCH RECIPES 72
DINNER RECIPES 96
SNACKS & DESSERTS RECIPES 113
21 DAY MEAL-PLAN 133
5 TRUTH PRACTICALLY EVERYBODY MAKES SIRTFOOD DIET 148

INTRODUCTION

Of the hundreds of millions of people to adopt this year's popularized diets, fewer than 1 percent will gain significant weight loss. Not only are they failing to make a difference in the bulge war, but they are doing nothing to stem the wave of chronic disease that has engulfed modern society.

We can live longer but don't live healthier. Staggeringly, the amount of time we spend in ill health has doubled from 20 to 40 percent over a mere ten years. It means we are now spending nearly 32 years of our lives in poor health. Just check out the stats. One in ten has diabetes right now, and another three are on the brink of getting it. At some stage in their lives, two out of every ve people will be diagnosed with cancer. If you see three women over fifty years old, one of them will have an osteoporotic fracture. And in the average time it takes you to read a single page of this book, a new case of Alzheimer's is going to develop and somebody is going to die of heart disease — and that's only in the USA.

"Dieting" was never our thing, for those reasons. That's until we discovered Sirtfoods, a new — and easy — revolutionary way to eat your way to weight loss and wonderful health.

What SIRTFOODS Are?

When we cut back on calories, this causes an energy shortage that stimulates what is known as the "skinny gene," causing a torrent of positive change. It puts the body in a kind of survival mode where fat is prevented from being processed, and normal growth processes are put on hold. Instead, the body is turning its attention to burning up its fat stores and flipping on powerful housekeeping genes that fix and rejuvenate our cells, effectively giving them a spring clean. The upshot is weight loss and heightened disease resistance.

Yet cutting calories, as many dieters know, comes at a cost. Reducing energy intake in the short term is causing hunger, irritability, fatigue, and muscle loss. Long-term restriction on calories is causing our metabolism to stagnate. This is the collapse of all calorie-restrictive diets and paves the way for a piling back on the weight. For these reasons, 99 percent of dietitians are doomed to long-term failure.

All this led us to ask a big question: is it possible to activate our thin gene somehow with all the wonderful bene ts that carry with all those disadvantages without having to stick to an extreme calorie limit?

Enter Sirtfoods, a collection of wonder-foods newly discovered. Sirtfoods are particularly rich in special nutrients that can cause the same skinny genes in our bodies when we eat them as calorie restriction does. Those genes are called sirtuins. In a landmark study in 2003, they first came to light when researchers discovered that resveratrol, a compound found in red grape skin and red wine, dramatically increased the yeast's lifespan.2 Resveratrol had the same effect on longevity as calorie restriction, but this was achieved without reducing energy intake.

Red wine was hailed as the original sirtfood with its rich resveratrol content, explaining the health bene ts associated with its consumption, and even why people who drink red wine gain less weight.5 Nevertheless, this is just the beginning of the Sirtfood tale.

The world of health research was at the cusp of something big with the discovery of resveratrol, and the pharmaceutical industry wasted no time jumping on board. Researchers have started screening thousands of different chemicals for their capacity to activate our sirtuin genes. This identified a number of natural plant compounds with significant sirtuin-activating properties, not just resveratrol. It was also found that a given food could contain a whole range of these plant compounds, which could function together to both assist absorption and enhance the sirtuin-activating effect of that food. This had been one of the great resveratrol puzzles. When drunk as part of red wine, scientists working with resveratrol frequently had to use much higher doses than we realize they provide a bene t.

Nevertheless, as well as resveratrol, red wine contains a number of other natural plant compounds, including large concentrations of piceatannol as well as quercetin, myricetin, and epicatechin, each of which has been shown to activate our sirtuin genes independently and, more importantly, to function in coordination.

The dilemma for the pharmaceutical industry is that they can not sell the next major breakthrough product as a collection of nutrients or foods. So instead, they invested hundreds of millions of dollars in the hopes of uncovering a Shangri-la pill to develop and conduct tests of synthetic compounds. Multiple studies of sirtuin-activating drugs for a multitude of chronic diseases are currently underway, as is the rest-ever FDA-approved trial to investigate whether the medicine can slow aging.

If experience has taught us something, it's that we shouldn't keep much hope for this synthetic ambrosia, as tantalizing as that might be. The pharmaceutical and health industries have continually attempted to imitate the bene ts of foods and diets by isolated nutrients and medications. And it has come up short time and again. Why wait 10-plus years for these so-called miracle drugs to be approved, and the unavoidable side effects they carry, because right now we have all the amazing bene ts available through the food we eat at our fingertips?

And while the pharmaceutical industry is chasing a drug-like magic bullet aggressively, we need to retrain our attention on dieting. Because at the same time, those efforts were underway, the nutritional science environment was also changing, posing some of its own big questions. Red wine on one side, were there other high-level foods of these special nutrients able to activate our sirtuin genes? And if so, what effects have they had on triggering fat loss and fighting disease?

WHAT IS THE SIRTFOOD DIET?

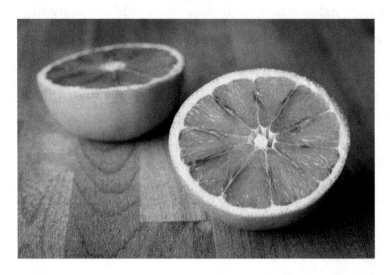

This Diet relies on research sirtuins (SIRTs), a set of seven proteins utilized from the human anatomy that's been proven to modulate various purposes, including inflammation, metabolism, and life span.

Certain Natural plant chemicals could possibly find a way to grow the degree of those proteins inside the human anatomy, and foods containing them are known"sirtfoods."

The Diet blends sirtfoods and calorie limitation, both of which may possibly cause the human body to generate high degrees of sirtuins.

The Sirtfood Diet publication comprises meal plans and recipes to follow along; however, there are lots of additional Sirtfood Diet recipe books out there.

The Diet's founders claim that after a Sirtfood Diet can cause accelerated body weight loss while maintaining muscles and protecting you in chronic illness.

Once You've finished the dietary plan, you're invited to keep on adding sirtfoods and also the diet signature green juice to your normal diet.

Thus Much, there aren't any persuasive signs that the Sirtfood Diet features a more favorable impact on weight loss than every other calorie-restricted diet regime.

Along with Although a number of those foods have healthy properties, there have yet to be any longterm human studies to ascertain if eating a diet full of sirtfoods has some concrete health benefits.

Nonetheless, the Sirtfood Diet publication reports the outcomes of a pilot study conducted with both the writers and between 3 9 participants in their exercise center. Nevertheless, the consequences of the study appear never to have already been released somewhere else.

To get 1 week, the participants followed the diet and worked out each day. At the close of the week, the participants lost an average of 5 pounds (3.2 kg) and claimed even gained muscle tissue.

Yet These outcomes are hardly surprising. Restricting your own calorie intake to 1000 calories and exercising at the exact same period will almost always trigger weight loss.

No matter This type of fast fat reduction is neither true nor long-term, which analysis failed to accompany participants following the initial week to determine whether they attained some of the weight , and this is an average of the situation.

When Your own body is energy-deprived, it melts away its catastrophe energy stores, or glycogen, along with burning off muscle and fat.

Each Molecule of glycogen necessitates 3--4 atoms of water to bestow. Whenever your body melts away glycogen, then it eliminates the water too. It's referred to as"water."

The very first week of extreme calorie limit, just about one-fifth of those fat loss arises from fat, whereas one other two-thirds stems out of water, glycogen, and muscle.

When your calories grow, the own body accomplishes its own glycogen stores, and also, the weight comes back again.

Regrettably, Such a calorie restriction may also cause the human body to reduce its metabolism, which makes it need fewer calories every day for energy compared to previously.

Additionally, it Is very likely that diet might help you drop a couple of pounds at the start, although it is going to probably return once the diet has ended.

As Much as preventing illness, three weeks might be long enough to own some measurable long-term effects.

The flip side, adding sirtfoods to a routine diet within the longterm, might just be a fantastic idea. However, in this circumstance, you may too, bypass the diet and begin doing this today.

IS IT REALLY EFFECTIVE?

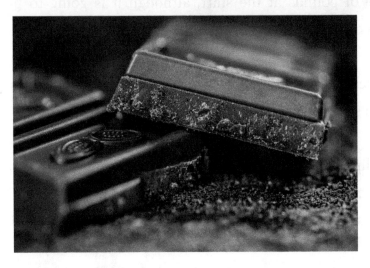

Thus Much, there aren't any persuasive signs that the Sirtfood Diet features a more favorable impact on weight loss than every other calorie-restricted diet regime.

Along with Although a number of those foods have healthy properties, there have yet to be any longterm human studies to ascertain if eating a diet full of sirtfoods has some concrete health benefits.

Nonetheless, the Sirtfood Diet publication reports the outcomes of a pilot study conducted with both the writers and between 3 9 participants in their exercise center. Nevertheless, the consequences of the study appear never to have already been released somewhere else.

To get 1 week, the participants followed the diet and worked out each day. At the close of the week, the participants lost an average of 5 pounds (3.2 kg) and claimed even gained muscle tissue.

Yet These outcomes are hardly surprising. Restricting your own calorie intake to 1000 calories and exercising at the exact same period will almost always trigger weight loss.

No matter This type of fast fat reduction is neither true nor long-term, which analysis failed to accompany participants following the initial week to determine whether they attained some of the weight , and this is an average of the situation.

When Your own body is energy-deprived, it melts away its catastrophe energy stores, or nourishment, along with burning off muscle and fat.

Each Molecule of glycogen necessitates 3--4 molecules of water to bestow. Whenever your body melts away glycogen, then it eliminates the water too. It's referred to as"water."

The very first week of extreme calorie limit, just about one-fifth of those fat loss arises from fat, whereas one other two-thirds stems out of water, glycogen, and muscle.

When your calories grow, the own body interrupts its own glycogen stores, and also, the weight comes back again.

Regrettably, Such a calorie restriction may also cause the human body to reduce its metabolism, inducing need fewer calories every day for energy compared to previously.

Additionally, it Is very likely that diet might help you drop a couple of pounds at the start, although it is going to probably return once the diet has ended.

As Much as preventing illness, three weeks might be long enough to own some measurable long-term effects.

The flip side, adding sirtfoods to a routine diet within the longterm, might just be a fantastic idea. However, in this circumstance, you may too, bypass the diet and begin doing this today.

This diet might help you drop weight since it's low in carbs; however, the weight is very likely to reunite once the diet ends. The diet plan is too short of owning a longterm influence on your own wellbeing.

What Does this involve?

The Sirtfood Diet contains 2 stages. About all the first few days, you just drink three 'sirt juices' and also have just one meal (full of 1000 calories each day). Over the subsequent four days, you are allowed two sirt juices along with 2 meals per day (full of 1,500 calories per day). Then you advance to the much easier phase 2, together with one juice along with also three'balanced' meals, in thoughtful portion sizes, daily.

Can be It successful for fat loss?

Now you Should shed weight only because you are eating more calories, notably at phase one. Really, you might burn up fat faster with this specific diet compared to with any 'aged calorie-restricted' plan, and also you may feel fitter. In terms of the writers' assert that this diet is 'scientifically proven to get rid of 7lb in a week'...

Well, It's well worth noting so much the dietary plan has just been tested to 40 healthy, highly motivated human guinea pigs in an upmarket gymnasium in London's Knightsbridge. The researchers lost a mean of 7lb per week while revealing increases in muscular density and energy. But given that the calorie restrictions of the very first week, fat loss could simply be caused by the extreme decrease in calories.

The verdict

Further studies are required to spot the longterm effect on waistlines -- and also standard health -- and also to check if sirt dieters maintain off the pounds more efficiently than they might on other diet plans. We do not yet understand exactly what, if any, impact the accession of sirtfoods into our daily diet actually is wearing our burden reduction.

Along with Will, anybody has the ability to stay to the monotony of juices and also limit themselves into foods among the list (and be more delighted to ditch their usual cuppa for green-tea) forever? In terms of the news headlines which suggest you may enjoy chocolate brown and red wine onto this particular diet well, the truth is, it is maybe not really a green light to eat up mountains of !

Cutting Calories will consistently provide results

In case You possess the financing, the tendency, and the gut because of it, I am pretty sure it'll 'work' for some degree at the brief term, if just because it's a highly effective approach to restrict calories. And chocolate and wine aside, the list chiefly is made up of those most foods dietitians and nutritionists urge for Goodhealth (think fresh fruit and veg!)) .

Whether or not It works nicely enough to allow it to stand out apart from the tens of thousands of weight loss plans which have trodden this tired course before additionally remains to be viewed. It's likely Goggins and Matten will end up best selling diet writers. However, I guess the mega-bucks will truly flow after the pharmaceutical industry manages to make sirtuin modulators which we're able to soda, therefore there will be no requirement to down still another carrot smoothie.

HOW TO ADHERE TO THE SIRTFOOD DIET

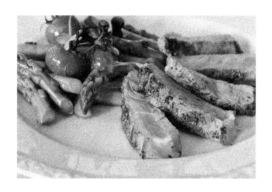

The Sirtfood Diet contains two stages that survive a total of 3 weeks. From then on, you're able to carry on "sirtifying" your daily diet by adding many sirtfoods as you possibly can on meals. The Special recipes for both of these stages can be located in The Sirtfood Diet publication, which has been compiled by the diet founders. You will have to get it to adhere to along with the diet program.

The foods Are filled with sirtfoods; however, do comprise other ingredients besides only the "high 20 sirtfoods."

The majority of The components and sirtfoods are a breeze to discover.

But, Three of those signature ingredients demanded both of these stages -- matcha green tea extract powder, lovage, and buckwheat -- Maybe costly or difficult to get.

A big part of the diet plan is its own green juice, which You ought to produce your self between you and a few times each day. You'll Need a Juicer (a blender won't work) and also a kitchen , whilst the ingredients are all Recorded by weight. The recipe is below:

Sirtfood Green Juice

- 75 g (2.5 ounces) lettuce
- 30 g (1 ounce) arugula (rocket)
- 5 g parsley
- Two celery sticks
- 1 cm (0.5 in) ginger
- Half of per green apple
- half a lemon
- half per teaspoon matcha green tea

Juice Ingredients aside from your own green tea extract powder and lemon and put them in a glass. Juice the lemon hand, then stir fry either lemon juice and green tea powder in your juice.

Period One

The Very First Phase lasts 7 days also involves calorie limitation and a lot of green juice. It's meant to jumpstart your weight-loss reduction and promised to simply help you to lose 5 pounds (3.2 kg) in 7 days.

The very initial 3 days of period one, calories are confined to 1000 calories. You beverage three green juices every day and something meal. Daily you'll be able to pick from recipes from the publication, which involve sirtfoods like the most important portion of the meal.

Meal Examples comprise miso-glazed lettuce, the sirtfood omelet, or even a shrimp stirfry with buckwheat noodles.

On days 4--7 phase one, calories are raised to 1,500. This consists of two green juices every day and 2 sirtfood-rich meals that you are able to select from the publication.

Period Two

Period two Lasts for 2 or three weeks. Throughout this "care" period, you should keep to gradually drop weight.

There Was No particular calorie limitation for this particular period. As an alternative, you eat three meals high of sirtfoods plus also one green juice daily. The meals are chosen in recipes given in the publication.

Subsequent to the Diet

You will Repeat both of these stages as frequently as desired for additional weight reduction.

But, You're encouraged to keep on "sirtifying" your daily diet after completing those periods by incorporating sirtfoods consistently to meals.

You will find An assortment of all Sirtfood Diet books which can be full of meals full of sirtfoods. It is possible to even incorporate sirtfoods on your diet plan for a bite or in recipes that you use.

In Addition, You're invited to keep on drinking the green juice daily.

In this Manner, the Sirtfood Diet becomes a lifestyle change than the usual onetime diet.

Can It be Sustainable and Healthy?

Sirtfoods Are nearly all nutritious choices and might even cause a few health benefits due to their anti-inflammatory or anti-inflammatory properties.

Yet Eating a small number of especially well-balanced meals can't meet most of your system's nutrient needs.

The Sirtfood Diet is restrictive and will be offering no clear, exceptional health and fitness benefits over another sort of diet plan.

Moreover, Eating just 1000 calories is, on average, not recommended with no oversight of a doctor. Eating 1,500 calories a day is too restrictive for a lot of men and women.

The Diet additionally requires drinking to three green juices every day. Even though juices can become quite a very good supply of minerals and vitamins, they're also a supply of sugars and also comprise nearly none of the nutritious fiber which whole vegetables and fruits do.

What is More, sipping juice all through the entire afternoon is a terrible idea for the blood glucose along with your own teeth. Perhaps not Obviously, since the diet is indeed restricted in food and calorie choice, it really is most likely deficient in protein, minerals, and vitamins, particularly throughout the first period. Because of the minimal-carb levels, along with restrictive eating food choices, this diet might be tricky to stick to for the full 3 weeks.

Insert That into the high first expenses of needing to buy a juicer, even the publication along with certain infrequent and costly ingredients, in addition to enough timing costs of organizing specific juices and meals; also, this particular diet gets laborious and disheartening for lots of men and women.

We Regularly find out about the benefits of drinking green tea extract, and it's really correct; this beverage includes a massive selection of useful benefits. Drinking only 1 cup every day can truly allow you to emotionally and physically, and below are a few of the most usual advantages of green tea extract.

1. Green Tea Extract Helps the Human Brain

It is Not about the physical advantages since green tea extract can allow one to feel faster and start to become emotionally fatigued. Individuals who study that a lot should consider buying matcha green tea extract since they'll discover that drinking green tea on a regular basis permits them to are better and work more efficiently.

2. It calms Your Metabolism

People Looking to shed weight frequently find a small benefit in drinking green tea extract concerning fostering your own metabolic process. Which usually means they will burn up fat quicker, and also provided that the remainder of these diet plan is a healthier and balanced yet, they'll be in a position to burn up calories and fat and reduce the extra weight they are attempting to knock out.

3. It Can Help Maintain Cancers Off

Even though there are lots of healthful meals and drinks that could help keep away cancer green tea, green tea is just another you can drink so as to keep much healthier. Polyphenols that are available in green tea extract is traditionally considered to help prevent cancer growth and dispersing in your system. It does so by preventing the cells from copying and growing as fast.

4. It frees Your Skin wholesome

In case You are attempting to slow the aging processor be certain your face does not develop wrinkles too fast; green tea extract may be just the thing that will assist you. While drinking a lot, it could irritate you, meaning it is crucial that you simply drink water; also, in the event that you'd like the skin to remain healthy daily, 23 glasses of green tea extract can boost your general skin health.

5. It may withstand Different ailments

In addition to keeping away cancer, green tea comprises free radicals that help keep different diseases off. This can involve diabetes, arthritis, as well as different bone-related disorders. So as to gain out of this, you also should begin drinking green tea extract just as early as you possibly can and drink it on a normal basis.

6. It may Reduce Cholesterol

When People today grow old, certainly one of the principal issues they whine of is elevated cholesterol. The doctors and other caregivers, in many cases, are telling us exactly what we will need to perform as a way to manage a wholesome cholesterol level enhance the way you live. Green tea extract can assist with this, even though you ought to avoid unhealthy foods and exercise regularly too.

7. Greentea Enhances Your Memory

In case You also end up forgetting things readily, a couple of glasses of green tea extract weekly may be just the thing that you should help the human mind improve also to assist you to remember things. This helps at work while analyzing with life in general, and you're able to impress people with how well it is possible to remember modest information!

SIRTFOOD DIET -- PHASE ONE

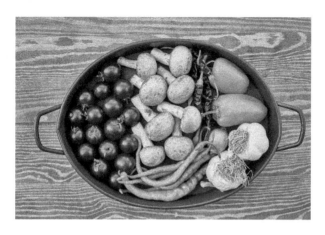

The Plan asserts that eating particular foods can trigger your "lean receptor" pathway and possess you losing seven pounds in 7 days. Foods such as ginseng, dark chocolate, and milk contain a natural compound called polyphenols, which mimic the results of fasting and exercise. Strawberries, red onions, cinnamon, and garlic will also be powerful sirtfoods. These foods can activate the sirtuin pathway to help activate weight reduction. The science seems appealing; however, in reality, there is very little research to back up these claims. Plus, the guaranteed speed of weight reduction from the very first week is quite quick and perhaps not in accord with the National Institute of Health's safe fat loss recommendations of a couple of pounds each week.

The Diet includes 2 stages:
- Stage one endures for 2 days. For the initial 3 days, you only drink three sirtfood green juices along with something meal full of sirtfoods for an overall total of 1000 calories. On days four through seven, you just beverage two juices and 2 meals for a total of 1,500 calories.
- Stage 2 is really a 14day maintenance program, though it's created to your shed weight steadily (perhaps not maintain your present weight). Daily is composed of three balanced sirtfood meals plus also one green juice.

Later Those 3 weeks, you are invited to keep on eating a diet full of sirtfoods and drinking with a green juice each day. It's possible to discover several sirtfood cookbooks on the web and also recipes to the sirtfood internet site . 1 green juice recipe entirely on the sirtfood internet site is made up of a combination of spinach and other leafy greens, celery, carrot, green apple, ginger, lemon juice, and matcha. Buckwheat and lovage may also be things that can be advocated for use on your green juice. The diet urges that juices need to be drawn up in a juicer, so perhaps not really a blender, so that it tastes better.

Now you Absolutely will need to plan and also have access to this ingredient that is recommended in order to correctly stick to this diet program. You can also have to put money into an adequate juicer that can set you back no less than 100. Form completely free recipes which can be found on the site, you could require to put money into a few of The Sirtfood Diet cookbooks.

Seasonality Of components makes it somewhat tough to have kale and tomatoes times of this season. Additionally, it is hard to follow along if traveling at social events and feeding on a family with young children.

The Diet cuts numerous food collections, and also it is limiting. Dairy foods that give a range of crucial nutritional elements, including several that a lot of folks lack, is not advocated on the strategy. What's more, the polyphenol-rich food matcha frequently contains lead from the tea leaves that will be potentially dangerous for your health, particularly when taken regularly. Additionally, it includes a robust and bitter flavor, as does 85% black chocolate, and this can also be suggested.

Sirtfood Nutrition Strategies

When You abide by the Sirtfood daily diet, you are going to start out with phase one --that lasts for 2 days. Throughout the first 3 days of this daily diet plan, you're beverage three Sirtfood juices and also consume just one Sirtfood-rich meal to get a regular total of 1000 calories. On times per week through seven, you'll have 1,500 total calories, then drink two juices and then eat just two healthy Sirtfood-rich meals. This finishes phase 1).

Phase 2 lasts a fortnight and enables one to eat three balanced Sirtfood-rich meals plus also one green juice each day. Once phase 2 is finished, you are going to adhere to a more ordinary manner of eating--however, are invited to include sirtuin-activating foods to routine meal plans. It's possible to re-enter phase 1 and two almost any moment you will need to shed weight or excess fat.

Foods You May Eat
You will probably wish to get a juicer when after the Sirtfood diet. These foods and beverages are supported:
- green juices (including matcha green tea extract, lovage, and buckwheat)
- green tea
- Coffee
- Cocoa powder
- dark chocolate
- Beef
- Kale
- Onions
- Parsley
- Coffee

- coconut oil
- Crimson chicory
- noodle berry
- berries
- berries
- Walnuts
- Eggs
- Bacon
- Turkey
- Sea-food
- Whole Grain pitas
- Cheese
- Hummus
- Buckwheat noodles
- Dark Wine

Can The Diet Function?

One Reason you will pro lose some pounds in the event that you adhere to that the Sirtfood diet accurately is since you'll lose calories (at least phase 1) to 1,000 to 1,500 calories every day, that can be an almost sure-fire method to lose weight reduction

The main point is that you never need to eat sirtuin-activating foods to lose weight (simply lowering your current calories have to have the desired effect), nearly all Sirtfoods are more healthy, seem to reduce disease risks, and also help with healthy weight control.

How do I prepare for your initial Phase of this daily diet

It is The clear question: should sirtuins are therefore game-changing, why are not pharmaceutical and nutritional supplement organizations attempting to distill them to pill form? Short answer: since the mechanics whereby they operate are still not fully known, meaning supps won't necessarily function absorbed from your system as the organic forms.

"In supplement type, it is poorly consumed by The entire human anatomy, however in its own normal food matrix of red wine, its bioavailability (just how much your human body is able to utilize) is sixfold greater. We believe it's much better to eat up a vast selection of these nutritional elements from the kind of pure whole foods, where they revolve together with the countless additional natural bioactive plant compounds that act responsibly to enhance our wellness." In different word seats, instead of simply popping a pill.

SIRTFOOD DIET -- PHASE TWO

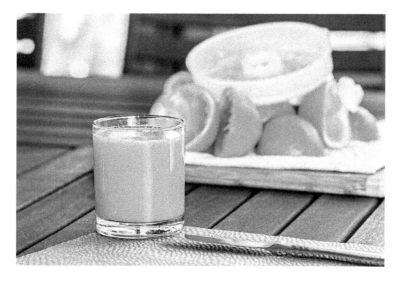

Minerals And vitamins to which women may possibly require supplements contain iron, calcium, Vitamins B6, B12, and vitamin D. Men, but need to pay attention to magnesium, fiber, Vitamins b 9 Vitamin C and E.

This Premise pertains to weight loss diet plans too. Men's and women's nutrition requirements impact which weight loss diet plans are far better for each gender.

In case You are like a lot of people, you've seen a remarkable quantity of fat loss programs and styles come and go; just about most of them have their own merits, and virtually most they work

-- temporarily. Weight control and health care professionals assert nearly unanimously that the age-old, tried and true blend of good nutrition and regular exercise may be the ideal approach to effortlessly eliminate weight and keep it off.

To get A number folks, it might well not be that hard to shed weight or maintain a healthy weight; however, the Sirtfood diet may help individuals who find themselves struggling. However, think about blending the Sirtfood diet exercise, can it be wise to prevent the exercise or present it when you've begun diet?

The SirtDiet Basics

Together with An estimated 650 million obese adults internationally, it is vital that you come across nutritious eating and workout regimes that can be attainable, do not dissuade one of all you like, and also do not ask that you exercise weekly. The Sirtfood diet really does only that. The notion is that food items are going to occupy the'skeletal gene' pathways that usually are actuated by exercise and fasting. The fantastic thing is that food and beverage, such as black chocolate and red wine, also contain compounds called polyphenols which trigger the enzymes which mimic the results of fasting and exercise.

Exercise Throughout the first couple of weeks

The very first fourteen days of the dietary plan where your calorie consumption is paid off, it'd be sensible to discontinue or lose exercise while the human body adjusts to fewer calories. Listen to your own body, and in the event that you're feeling tired or consume less energy than normal, do not workout. As an alternative, make certain you remain centered on the fundamentals that are pertinent to a wholesome lifestyle, such as adding sufficient daily degrees of fiber, fruit and protein, and veggies.

Once The diet gets to be a method of life

When You really do exercise, it is crucial to eat up protein an hour or so after your work out. Protein fixes muscles after exercise, reduces soreness, and also may aid recovery. There are certainly a number of recipes, including protein that'll probably be perfect for post-exercise ingestion, like the sirt chili con Carne or perhaps the garlic poultry and tofu salad. If you'd like something lighter, you can try out the sirt sour smoothie and then put in some protein powder for extra benefit. The form of workout you do would be right down for you personally; however, workouts in the home will make it possible for you to decide when to exercise, the sorts of exercises which suit you personally and also, therefore, are easy and short.

The Sirtfood diet is an excellent means to alter your diet plan, drop weight, and feel much healthier. The very first couple of weeks can challenge you; however, it is crucial that you assess which foods are best to eat and delicious recipes suit you personally. Be kind to your self in the very first couple of weeks while the system adjusts and requires action easy if you opt to accomplish it whatsoever. If you're already somebody would you intense or moderate exercise; then it could possibly be that you're able to keep on as normal or even manage your fitness regimen in accordance with the shift in diet. Just like with any diet and exercise varies, it's about the person and how much you'll be able to push your self.

The Sirtfood Bird's-Eye Chilies comprise the significant sirtuin-activating nutrition Luteolin and Myricetin.

Earth's Eye Chilies(some times known as 'Thai chilies') are among the very best 20 Sirtfoods and look frequently from the recipe segments (here and here) with this site. If you aren't utilized to hot food, then it's advised that you begin with half of a chili amount mentioned within the recipe, in addition to deseeding your chili prior usage. It's possible to adjust the heat for a taste all through your diet plan.

Chili Launched from the Americas, and it has been part of this diet since 7500 BC. Explorer Christopher Columbus brought it back to Spain from the 15 century, and its farming spread quickly throughout the remainder of the earth. Its pungent heat was created as a plant defense system to cause vexation and discourage predators from feasting about it, yet many individuals enjoy adding it for their eating routines.

There Are over 200 forms, colored such a thing out of yellowish to green to reddish to dark, and varying in heat from slightly hot into mouth-blisteringly hot.

Earth's - Eye Chilies boast far greater sirtuin-activating credentials compared to the milder regular chilies which are additionally utilized.

Earth's -Eye Chilies are famous for weight loss reduction qualities. They are able to play an integral part in increasing the metabolic process of your system by boosting your body's temperature. Faster metabolic rate, good nourishment, and waste expulsion may reduce the odds of fat accumulation within your system.

The Chemical compound found in Bird's-Eye chili, which leads from the burning sensation, is named Capsaicin. The impacts of the chemical may vary among humans. But most frequent is that a burning sensation of the throat, mouth, and stomach about intake.

It does Not simply heat of chilies, however, the direction that they boost the flavors of different ingredients

Everything You Need to expect from the Second phase

In case You are a convert to green tea, and then congratulations, you'll be reaping the advantages of the Extra Ordinary sirtuins seen in green tea extract. You'll locate fat comes more readily, along with a revitalized soul and luminous skin.

Exactly why Is drinking green tea extract, therefore, vital?

Green Tea is the sole supply of a few of the strongest sirtuin bioactive, catechin. Catechins are so potent that just a little volume, one small cup, also activates fat metabolism also reduces oxidative stress.

- Appetite-suppressant

Together with A cup or two of green tea extract in you. You truly see the gap concerning the urge to eat. You ought to discover that you never consider food between meals.

- Slightly of caffeine

A Cup of green tea extract contains about a quarter of that caffeine you'd see in a cup of java or half of the caffeine you'd see in a cup of green tea. This caffeine is simply enough to unite with the catechins to truly have an even more effective Fat Burning effect. This could be the best means to convert fat into muscle.

- More energy

Hard To measure, however, absolutely there, the more catechins provide you only a modest all-natural buzz, which makes starting your afternoon a bit simpler.

- Cumulative effect

The Power of green tea keeps on two glasses of green tea extract is much far better compared to 1 cup, so three cups are far better than just two cups. Actually, you're able to get right up to four your SIRT 5 a day out of drinking green tea extract if you've got four or cups.

- Zero-calorie

Green Tea is obviously fat-free. It will not require sugar sweetener and provides you energy minus calories.

Here Are our best five most useful Sirtfoods for Goodhealth.

Dark Coffee

This Yummy cure keeps the heart fit and modulates blood pressure. Full of antioxidants, dark-chocolate spikes growing older and also combat free radicals. Additionally, it reinforces the body's immune mechanisms and wards away infections. Even the flavanols in chocolate can improve blood flow and reduce cognitive damage.

Green Tea

Loaded With antioxidants and cancer-fighting chemicals, green tea extract is perhaps one of the very effective all-natural remedies available on the market. This drink is produced of the dried leaves of the Camellia sinensis plant, which has been proven effective against pancreatic cancer, lung cancer, pancreatic cancer, diabetes, and prostate cancer. Green tea reduces cardiovascular disease risk, reduces cholesterol, also protects against stroke. Its weight reduction benefits are copied by mathematics fiction.

Blueberries

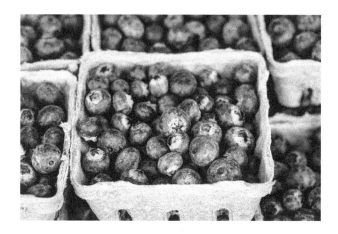

Blueberries Are a superb source when vitamin C, vitamin K, manganese, copper, and fiber. Additionally, they possess the greatest antioxidant content of most berries. These hot Sirtfoods boost resistance and neutralize the free radicals, which may damage cell structures. Low in carbs and calories, they are best for dieters. Recent studies imply that blueberries can help lessen abdominal fat and risk factors for metabolic syndrome. Full of calcium, they additionally strengthen your muscles and protect against osteoporosis.

Capers

Capers Boast strong anti-inflammatory effects, supplying a cocktail of vitamins, minerals, minerals, and antioxidants. They've just 2 3 calories per 100g and offer considerable amounts of potassium, calcium, vitamin K, riboflavin, iron, aluminum, and phytonutrients. Quercetin and rutin, the crucial antioxidants within capers, have strong analgesic, anti-bacterial, and anti-carcinogenic properties. Rutin helps treat and prevent psoriasis, improves flow, and reduces bad cholesterol levels in obese patients. Quercetin inhibits tumor development and also promotes immune function. The perfect method to make use of capers is always adding them into salads, pasta, pasta, and casseroles.

Turmeric

This Spice was used since early times because of its curative properties. Curcumin, its ingredients, has been a potent antioxidant and anti-inflammatory agent. This naturally occurring chemical reduces inflammation in the human own body, which will help prevent diabetes, chronic pain, cancer, obesity, cardiovascular problems, and various degenerative ailments. Turmeric also enriches your body's antioxidant capacity, struggles free deep damage, also improves brain functioning. This really is among those very few foods comprising BDNF (brain-derived neurotrophic factor), a protein that leads to this growth, maturation, and survival of neural cells.

All these Will be the 5 most useful Sirtfoods; however, there are quite a few different Sirtfoods with recognized health benefits, like apples, carrot, citrus fruit, as well as pineapple. Redwine comprises sirtuin activators too. Your diet needs to also include things like olive oil, passionfruit, and onions that excite sirtuin cells and boast top antioxidant levels.

GETTING STARTED: GROCERY LIST

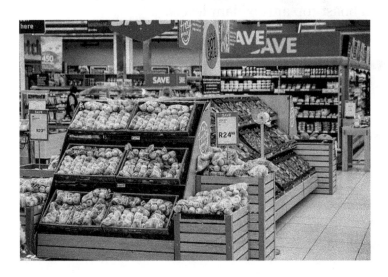

All these Would be the highest-rated 20 foods to get a Sirtfood-rich diet program and ways to incorporate them into your everyday meals.

Earth's - Eye Chili. Additionally sold as Thai chilies, they truly are stronger than ordinary chilies and packed with more nutritional elements. Utilize them to increase sour or sweet recipes.

Buckwheat. Technically a pseudo-grain: it's really a berry seed linked to rhubarb. Additionally, accessible noodle shape (like soba), but ensure that you're getting the wheat-free edition.

Capers. If you are wondering, then they are pickled flower buds. Sprinkle them a salad or roasted steaks.

Celery. The leaves and hearts would be the most healthful part, and thus do not throw them off if you are mixing a shakeup.

Chicory. Red is most beneficial, but yellowish works too. Include it into a salad.

Cocoa. The flavonol-rich type enhances blood pressure, blood glucose cholesterol, and control. Search to get a high proportion of cacao.

Coffee. Drink it shameful -- there are some signs that milk can lower the absorption of sirtuin-activating nutritional elements.

Extra Virgin Steak Oil. The extra-virgin type includes more Sirt benefits, and also a far more pleasing, flavor.

Green Tea or Matcha. Add a piece of lemon juice to raise the absorption of sirtuin-producing nutritional elements. Matcha is much better, but really go Japanese, not Chinese, in order to steer clear of potential lead contamination.

Kale. Includes huge levels of sirtuin-activating nutrition quercetin and kaempferol. Scrub it with coconut oil and lemon juice serve it as a salad.

Lovage. It is a herb. Grow your personal onto a window sill and throw it into stirfries.

Medjool Dates. They truly are a hefty 66 percent glucose, however in moderation -- do not raise glucose levels, also have been connected to reduced levels of diabetes and cardiovascular disease.

Parsley. More than only a garnish -- it's saturated in apigenin. Throw into a juice or smoothie for the complete benefit. Chicory Red is most beneficial, but yellowish functions fine. Throw it in a salad.

Red Onion. The reddish variety is healthier personally, and also sweet enough to eat raw. Stir it and put into a salad or eat it with a hamburger.

Red Wine. You've been aware of resveratrol: the fantastic news is that it is heat stable, which means it's possible to benefit from cooking together with it (in addition to glugging it directly). Pinot noir gets got the maximum content.

Rocket. One among the very least interfered-with salad greens out there. Drizzle it with olive oil.

Soy. Soybeans and miso are saturated in sirtuin activators. Include it into stirfries.

Strawberries. Though they are sweet, they simply comprise 1tsp of sugar per 100g -- and research suggests that they improve the ability to manage carbonated carbohydrates.

Turmeric. Evidence suggests the curcumin inside its anti-cancer properties. It's difficult for your human body to assimilate alone, however cooking it into fluid and including black pepper increases absorption.

Walnuts. Full of calories and fat, but well recognized in lessening metabolic disorder. Mash them up with skillet to get a sirt-flavored pesto.

Only A reminder of this scientific backdrop into the Sirtfood diet regime.

Sirtfoods Are the revolutionary way of triggering our sirtuin genes in the finest way possible. All these are the miracle foods, especially full of specific all-natural plant compounds, called polyphenols that possess the capability to trigger our sirtuin genes by changing them . Essentially, they mimic the results of exercise and fasting also, in doing this bring notable benefits by helping the system to better control glucose levels and burn fat, and build muscle and promote memory and health.

Because They're stationary plants also have developed an extremely complex stress-response system and also produce antioxidants to help them conform to the challenges in their own environment. Once we consume these plants, we additionally eat up these polyphenol nourishment. Their effect is strong: they trigger our very own inborn stress-response pathways.

Even though All plants possess stress-response techniques, just certain ones have grown to create impressive levels of sirtuin-activating polyphenols. All these plants are sirtfoods. Their discovery ensures instead of strict fasting regimens or tough exercise apps; there is presently a radically new means to trigger your sirtuin genes: eating a healthy diet loaded at sirtfoods. On top of that, the dietary plan involves putting (sirt)foods on your plate, so not carrying off them.

Would You Eat Meat About Your Sirtfood Diet?

The Answer can be a resounding, yes. The diet not just comprises ingesting a healthful part of beef, it urges that protein becomes a crucial addition within a Sirtfood-based diet plan to reap the most benefit in maintaining metabolic process and lessening the muscle imbalance common in many fat loss programs. It isn't just a beef heavy diet (we remember the awful breath out of the Atkins diet), it's actually very vegetarian friendly and caters to nearly everyone, and that's exactly what causes it to be sensible an alternative.

Leucine Is an amino acid found in protein that divides and actually enriches the action of Sirtfoods. This usually means that the perfect solution to consume Sirtfoods is by simply mixing them with chicken , beef, or alternative supply of leucine like eggs or fish.

Poultry Could be eaten (since it's a great source of protein, B vitamins, potassium, and phosphorous), also that red-meat (still another superb source of iron, protein, calcium, and vitamin b 12) might be consumed to 3 occasions (750g raw weight) weekly.

Foods Saturated in sirtuins (proteins which regulate cellular and metabolic purpose), can play a part in increasing our wellbeing, reducing inflammation, and also potentially helping in weight loss too. In the event you are worried this diet will soon be miserably restrictive, you are in fortune: those sirtuin-activating foods aren't simply full of good for you polyphenols, but they're also diverse, flavorful, also might be incorporated to your own diet in many of creative methods.

Sirtuin Activators and sirtfoods have become fresh to this science of nutrition. Now a 'sirtfood' is obviously a food packed in sirtuin activators. Vitamins were discovered over a hundred decades back, anti-oxidants 50 decades ago, and also sirtuin activators only over ten decades back.

The 1st sirtuin activator understood -- but the most effective known -- has been resveratrol, found in the skin of red grapes (and that's the reason why red wine is traditionally believed to continue to keep you healthy), pomegranates and Japanese knotweed.

Additional Sirtuin activators soon followed, like catechins (seen in green tea extract and also presumed to work with cancer cells) and epicatechins in cocoa powder (accountable for its health benefits of chocolates).

However, Research took away once the pharmaceutical giant GlaxoSmithKline bought the rights to generate artificial variations of resveratrol for 462 million. It hastens trial, such as a cancer treatment; however, the consequences weren't impressive. This season the organization announced it had ceased the research.

However, It today seems eating sirtfoods naturally full of sirtuin activators could be described as a much healthier, far better --

and cheaper -- alternative for supplements. It was considering the newest trials of sirtfoods as well as also the sirtfood dietary plan. Present results imply that sirtfoods target precisely the exact same path for reducing weight and staying fit since dietary restriction and physical exercise.

Resveratrol Seen in red wine might help counteract the unfavorable effect of elevated fat/high glucose diets-SirtFood Research

Red Wine fans have a new cause to observe. Researchers have located a brand new wellness advantage of resveratrol, that does occur naturally in blueberries, raspberries, mulberries, grape skins, and thus in crimson wine. Resveratol is recognized as a sirtuin activator.

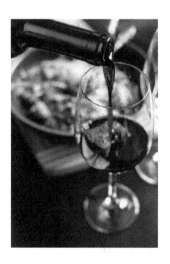

Even though Analyzing the results of resveratrol from the diet rhesus monkeys," Dr. J.P. Hyatt, an Associate Professor at Georgetown University, along with his group of investigators found a resveratrol supplement could counteract the bad effect of a superior fat/high sugar diet onto the thoracic muscles. In previous animal studies, resveratrol has shown to improve the life span of mice and slow down the onset of cardiovascular disease. In 1 study, it revealed the results of aerobic exercise mice, that have been fed with a superior fat/high sugar-free diet plan.

Even though These outcomes are reassuring, also there may possibly be a desire to keep on eating a superior fat/high sugar and just incorporate a glass of red wine or even a cup of fresh fruit to someone's daily ingestion, the investigators highlight that the value of a wholesome diet can't be overemphasized. However, for the time being, there is an additional reason to really have a glass of wine.

Decreasing The probability Of Persistent Disease-SirtFood Research

There Are growing signs that sirtuin activators can have a vast selection of health benefits in addition to building muscle and curbing desire. These generally include improving memory, so helping your human body control glucose levels, and clearing up the damage from free radical molecules, which could collect in cells and result in cancer and various other diseases.

'Substantial Observational evidence is present for its favorable outcomes of the intake of food and beverage full of sirtuin activators in diminishing risks of chronic illness.

Even though Sirtuin activators are observed throughout the plant kingdom, just certain veggies and fruits have large amounts to count since SirtfFoods. Examples include things like green tea extract, cocoa powder, and the Indian spice broccoli, garlic, onions, and pineapple.

Most Of those vegetables and fruit available in supermarkets, like avocados, berries, lettuce, carrots, kiwis, carrots, and pineapple, are now quite saturated in sirtuin activators. It will not signify they aren't worth eating, however, since they provide tons of different advantages.

The Beauty of having a diet packaged using SirtFoods is it can become significantly more elastic compared to other diet plans. You might only eat adding some SirtFoods ontop. Or you might ask them to in a concentrated manner as advocated from the SirtFood diet regime.

BREAKFAST RECIPES

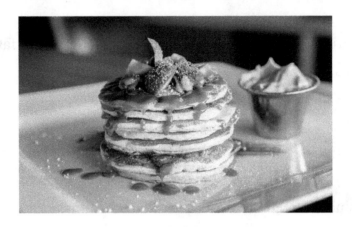

Mushroom Scramble Eggs

Ingredients

- 2 tbsp
- 1 teaspoon ground garlic
- 1 teaspoon mild curry powder
- 20g lettuce, approximately sliced
- 1 teaspoon extra virgin olive oil
- 1/2 bird's eye peeled, thinly chopped
- a couple of mushrooms, finely chopped
- 5g parsley, finely chopped
- *elective* Insert a seed mix for a topper plus Some Rooster Sauce for taste

Guidelines

- Mix the curry and garlic powder and then add just a little water till you've achieved a light glue.
- Steam the lettuce for two -- 3 minutes.
- Heat the oil in a skillet over a moderate heat and fry the chili and mushrooms 2-- three minutes till they've begun to soften and brown.
- Insert the eggs and spice paste and cook over moderate heat, then add the carrot and then proceed to cook over a moderate heat for a further minute. In the end, put in the parsley, mix well, and function.

Blue Hawaii Smoothie

Ingredients

- 2 tablespoons rings or approximately 4-5 balls
- 1/2 cup frozen tomatoes
- two Tbsp ground flaxseed
- 1/8 cup tender coconut (unsweetened, organic)
- few walnuts
- 1/2 cup fat-free yogurt
- 5-6 ice cubes
- dab of water

Guidelines

- Throw all of the ingredients together and combine until smooth. You might need to prevent and wake up to receive it combined smoothy or put in more water.

Turkey Breakfast Sausages

Ingredients

- 1 lb extra lean ground turkey
- 1 Tbsp EVOO, and a little more to dirt pan
- 1 Tbsp fennel seeds
- 2 teaspoon smoked paprika
- 1 teaspoon red pepper flakes
- 1 teaspoon peppermint
- 1 teaspoon chicken seasoning
- A couple of shredded cheddar cheese
- A couple of chives, finely chopped
- A few shakes garlic and onion powder
- Two spins of pepper and salt

Guidelines

- Pre Heat oven to 350F.
- Utilize a little EVOO to dirt a miniature muffin pan.

- Combine all ingredients and blend thoroughly.
- Fill each pit on top of the pan and then cook for approximately 15-20 minutes. Each toaster differs; therefore, when muffin fever is 165, then remove.

Banana Pecan Muffins

Ingredients
- 3 Tbsp butter softened
- 4 ripe bananas
- 1 Tbsp honey
- ⅛ cup OJ
- 1 teaspoon cinnamon
- 2 cups all-purpose pasta
- 2 capsules
- a couple of pecans, sliced
- 1 Tbsp vanilla

Guidelines

- Preheat the oven to 180°C/ / 350°F.
- Lightly grease the bottom and sides of the muffin tin, and then dust with flour.
- Dust the surfaces of the tin gently with flour then tap to eradicate any excess.

- Peel and insert the batter to a mixing bowl and with a fork, mash the carrots; therefore that you've got a combination of chunky and smooth, then put aside.
- Insert the orange juice, melted butter, eggs, vanilla, and spices and stir to combine.
- Roughly chop the pecans onto a chopping board, when using, then fold throughout the mix.
- Spoon at the batter 3/4 full and bake in the oven for approximately 40 minutes, or until golden and cooked through.

Banana And Blueberry Muffins - SRC

Ingredients

- 4 large ripe banana, peeled and mashed
- 3/4 cup of sugar
- 1 egg, lightly crushed
- 1/2 cup of butter, melted (and a little extra to dust the interiors of this muffin tin)
- 2 cups of blueberries (if they are suspended, do not defrost them. simply pop them into the batter suspended and)
- 1 teaspoon baking powder
- 1 teaspoon baking soda
- 1/2 teaspoon salt

- 1 cup of coconut bread
- 1/2 cup of flour (or 1-1;two cup bread)
- 1/2 cup applesauce
- dab of cinnamon

Guidelines

- Add mashed banana to a large mixing bowl.
- Insert sugar & egg and mix well.
- Add peanut butter and strawberries.
- Sift all the dry ingredients together, then add the dry ingredients into the wet mix and mix together lightly.
- Set into 12 greased muffin cups
- Bake for 20-30min in 180C or 350 F.

Morning Meal Sausage Gravy

Ingredients

- 1 lb sausage
- 2 cups 2 percent milk (complete is great also)
- 1/4 cup entire wheat bread
- salt and a Lot of pepper to flavor

Guidelines

- Cook sausage from skillet.
- Add flour and blend cook for about a minute.

- Insert two cups of milk.
- Whisk Whilst gravy thickens and bubbles.
- Add pepper and salt and keep to taste until flawless.
- Let stand a minute or so to ditch and function over several snacks.

Easy Egg-white Muffins

Ingredients

- Language muffin - I enjoy Ezekiel 7 grain
- egg-whites - 6 tbsp or two large egg whites
- turkey bacon or bacon sausage
- sharp cheddar cheese or gouda
- green berry
- discretionary - lettuce, and hot sauce, hummus, flaxseeds, etc.

Guidelines

- At a microwavable safe container, then spray entirely to stop the egg from adhering, then pour egg whites into the dish.
- Lay turkey bacon or bacon sausage paper towel and then cook .
- Subsequently, toast your muffin, if preferred.

- Then put the egg dish in the microwave for 30 minutes. Afterward, with a spoon or fork, then immediately flip egg within the dish and cook for another 30 minutes.
- Whilst dish remains hot sprinkle some cheese while preparing sausage.
- The secret is to get a paste of some kind between each coating to put up the sandwich together, i.e., a very small little bit of hummus or even cheese.

Sweet Potato Hash

Ingredients

- 1 Sweet-potato
- 1/2 red pepper, diced
- 3 green onions, peppermint
- leftover turkey, then sliced into bits (optional)
- 1 Tbsp of butter - perhaps a bit less (I never quantify)
- carrot powder - a few shakes
- Pepper - only a small dab to get a bit of warmth
- pepper and salt to flavor
- scatter of cheddar cheese (optional)

Guidelines

- Stab a sweet potato and microwave for 5 minutes.

- Remove from microwave, peel the skin off, and foliage.
- At a skillet, on medium-high warmth, place peppers and butter and sauté to get a few minutes.
- Insert potato bits and keep sautéing.
- Whilst sauté, add sweeteners, leafy vegetables, and green onions.
- Insert a dab of cheddar and Revel in!

Asparagus, Mushroom Artichoke Strata

Ingredients

- 1 little loaf of sourdough bread
- 4 challah rolls
- 8 eggs
- 2 cups of milk
- 1 teaspoon salt
- 1/4 teaspoon black pepper
- 1 cup Fontina cheese, cut into little chunks
- 1/2 cup shredded Parmesan cheese
- 1 Tbsp butter (I used jojoba)
- 1 teaspoon dried mustard
- 1/2 can of artichoke hearts, sliced
- 1 bunch green onions, grated
- 1 bunch asparagus, cut into 1-inch bits

- 1 10oz package of baby Bella (cremini) mushrooms, chopped

Guidelines

1. Clean mushrooms and slice and trim asparagus and cut in 1-inch pieces. Reserve in a bowl and scatter 1/2 teaspoon salt mixture.
2. Drain and dice 1/2 may or modest artichoke hearts.
3. Melt butter in a pan over moderate heat, also sauté the asparagus and mushrooms before the mushrooms start to brown, about 10 minutes.
4. Blend the artichoke core pieces into a bowl with all a mushroom/asparagus mix. Setaside.
5. Cut or split a tiny sourdough loaf into 1-inch bits. (My loaf was a little too small, therefore that I used 4 challah rolls too)
6. Grease a 9x13 inch baking dish and generate a base coating of bread at the dish. Spread 1/2 cup of Fontina cheese bread, at a coating, and disperse half an apple mixture on the cheese.
7. Lay-down a different layer of these vegetables and bread and high using a 1/2 cup of Fontina cheese.
8. Whisk together eggs, salt, milk, dry mustard, and pepper into a bowl and then pour the egg mixture on the vegetables and bread.

9. Cover the dish, and then simmer for 3 weeks.
10. Pre Heat oven to 375 degrees.
11. Eliminate the casserole from the fridge and let stand for half an hour.
12. Spread All the Parmesan cheese at a coating within the strata.
13. Bake in the preheated oven until a knife inserted near the border comes out clean, 40 to 45 minutes. Let stand 5 to 10 minutes before cutting into squares.

Egg White Veggie Wontons w/Fontina topped w/ crispy Prosciutto

Ingredients

- 1 cup egg whites
- butter
- fontina cheese
- mixed shredded cheddar cheese
- broccoli I utilized wheat, chopped bits
- tomatoes - diced
- salt and pepper
- prosciutto - two pieces

Guidelines

1. Remove Won Ton wrappers out of the freezer.
2. Pre Heat oven to 350.
3. Spray miniature cupcake tin with cooking spray.
4. After wrappers begin to defrost, peel off them carefully - apart, one at a time and press cupcake tin lightly.
5. I sliced the wrappers having a little bit of peanut butter. (optional)
6. set a chunk of cheese in every bottom.
7. Satisfy desired lettuce - I used pre-cooked broccoli bits and diced tomatoes.
8. Pour egg whites all toppings.
9. Sprinkle each with some of those shredded cheddar cheese.
10. Cook for approximately 15 minutes, but get started watching them afterward 10 - whenever they poof up - assess them poking the middle with a fork.
11. While eggs are cooking, then spray a sheet of foil with cooking spray and then put 2 pieces of prosciutto onto it and then cook at exactly the exact same period as the egg whites. After 8 minutes, then take and let sit once it cools it becomes crispy and chop and high eggs!

Crunchy and Chewy Granola

Ingredients

- Two 1/4 cup old-style yogurt
- 1 Tbsp flax seeds
- 1/4 tsp kosher salt
- 1/2 tsp cinnamon
- 1/4 ground ginger
- 1/2 cup honey
- two Tbsp packaged splendid brown-sugar
- 3/4 cup ounces raw peppers
- 1/2 cup sliced peppers
- 1/2 cup golden raisins
- 1/2 cup dried cranberries
- 1 Tbsp vanilla sugar to earn put a used vanilla bean in a full bowl of sugar and allow simmer for per month at icebox.

Guidelines
1. Pre Heat oven to 300.
2. Line baking sheet with parchment paper.
3. Mix 9 components together.
4. Insert 1 cup hot tap water, then mix together with hands and spread into a thin coating over a baking sheet.
5. Bake for 60 minutes, stirring 2-3 days, before turning black gold brown.
6. Remove from the oven and let cool.

7. Stir in dried fruit.
8. Dust with sugar.

Blueberry Pancakes

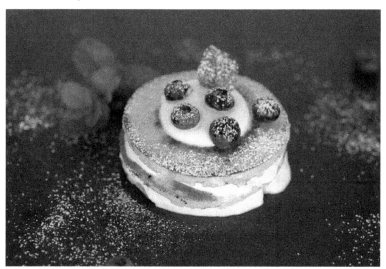

Ingredients

- 2 capsules
- 1 cup milk - then I used margarine
- 1 Tbsp vegetable oil
- 1.5 tsp butter melted, (and an additional piece of peanut butter to the pan)
- 1 1/4 cup All-purpose flour 3 tsp baking powder
- 3 tsp sugar
- 1/2 tsp salt
- 2 cups frozen blueberries

Guidelines

1. Put a nonstick griddle or a skillet over moderate heat.
2. Independent eggs yolks and whites, moving whites to some medium mixing bowl.
3. Whisk functions well with milk, butter, and oil.
4. Gradually fold dry ingredients to liquid with a wooden spoon.
5. In yet another bowl, sift together dry skin.
6. Working with an electric beater, whip egg whites until frothy.
7. Pour egg whites into the batter until just combined (small bumps of eggwhite are fine).
8. When skillet is hot, brush the skillet with melted butter.
9. Pour 1/4 cup batter onto the skillet for each pancake, leaving space .
10. Top each pancake using 5 6 blueberries, even if using.
11. When bubbles form inside the batter, then flip the pancake.
12. Keep on cooking until golden at the ground, about two minutes.
13. Drink instantly.

Power Balls

Ingredients

- 1 cup old fashion ginger, dried (I've used apple cinnamon-flavored oats also)
- 1/4 cup quinoa cooked using 3/4 cup orange juice
- 1/4 cup shredded unsweetened coconut
- 1/3 cup dried cranberry/raisin blend
- 1/3 cup dark chocolate chips
- 1/4 cup slivered almonds
- 1 Tbsp reduced-fat peanut butter

Guidelines

1. Cook quinoa in orange juice. Bring to boil and simmer for approximately 1-2 minutes. Let cool.
2. Combine chilled quinoa and the remaining ingredients into a bowl.
3. With wet hands and combine ingredients and roll in golden ball sized chunks.
4. Set at a Tupperware and set in the refrigerator for two weeks until the firm.

Cinnamon Crescent Rolls

Ingredients

- 2 cans refrigerated crescent rolls
- 1 stick butter, softened
- 1/2 cup brown or white sugar
- 1 tbsp cinnamon
- Glaze
- 1/2 cup powdered sugar
- 1 tsp vanilla
- 2 tbsp milk

Guidelines

1. Heat oven to 350°F.
2. In a small bowl, combine sugar, butter, and cinnamon; beat until smooth.
3. Separate dough into rectangles.
4. Spread each rectangle about two tbsp cinnamon butter mix.
5. Roll-up starting at the broadest side, as you'll ordinarily do to crescent rolls. Firmly press ends to seal.
6. Put each cinnamon filled crescent roll on a parchment lineup baking sheet. *Be sure that you line the cookie sheet, or that you might have a large mess after *
7. Bake for 10 to 15 minutes or until golden brown.

8. In a small bowl, combine all glaze ingredients, adding enough milk for desired drizzling consistency. Drizzle over hot rolls.

Fresh fruit Pizza

Ingredients

- 4 crescent rolls (Rolled-out and poked with a fork)
- Two spoonfuls of moderate Cream-cheese
- 1 teaspoon of sugar
- 1 teaspoon Vanilla extract
- Handful berries - chopped (You Can easily utilize lemon or blueberries)
- Sliced almonds

Guidelines

1. Place crescent rolls nonstick pan and then poke a few times with a fork. Cook at 375 for approximately 14 minutes. Let cool.
2. At a bowl, combine cream , Vanilla infusion & sugar stir with a spoon.
3. Spread onto crescent rolls, then add almonds and fruit.
4. I sprinkled a bit more sugar at the top after!

71

LUNCH RECIPES

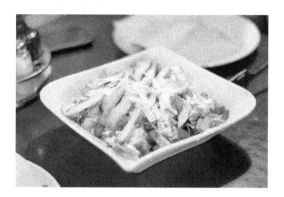

Sticky Chicken Water Melon Noodle Salad

Ingredients

- 2 pieces of skinny rice noodles
- 1/2 Tbsp sesame oil
- 2 cups Water Melon
- Head of bib lettuce
- Half of a Lot of scallions
- Half of a Lot of fresh cilantro
- 2 skinless, boneless chicken breasts
- 1/2 Tbsp Chinese five-spice
- 1 Tbsp extra virgin olive oil
- two Tbsp sweet skillet (I utilized a mixture of maple syrup using a dash of Tabasco)
- 1 Tbsp sesame seeds

- a couple of cashews - smashed
- Dressing - could be made daily or 2 until
- 1 Tbsp low-salt soy sauce
- 1 teaspoon sesame oil
- 1 Tbsp peanut butter
- Half of a refreshing red chili
- Half of a couple of chives
- Half of a couple of cilantro
- 1 lime - juiced
- 1 small spoonful of garlic

Guidelines
1. At a bowl, then completely substituting the noodles in boiling drinking water. They are going to soon be carried out in 2 minutes.
2. On a big sheet of parchment paper, then throw the chicken with pepper, salt, and also the five-spice.
3. Twist over the newspaper, subsequently celebration and put the chicken using a rolling pin.
4. Place into the large skillet with 1 Tbsp of olive oil, turning 3 or 4 minutes, until well charred and cooked through.
5. Drain the noodles and toss with 1 Tbsp of sesame oil onto a sizable serving dish.
6. Place 50% the noodles into the moderate skillet, stirring frequently until crispy and nice.

7. Eliminate the Watermelon skin, then slice the flesh to inconsistent balls and then increase the platter.
8. Reduce the lettuces and cut into small wedges and also half of a whole lot of leafy greens and scatter the dish.
9. Place another 1 / 2 the cilantro pack, the soy sauce, coriander, chives, peanut butter, and a dab of water, 1 teaspoon of sesame oil and the lime juice, then mix till smooth.
10. Set the chicken back to heat, garnish with all the sweet skillet (or my walnut syrup mixture), and toss with the sesame seeds.
11. Pour the dressing on the salad toss gently with fresh fingers until well coated, then add crispy noodles and then smashed cashews.
12. Blend chicken pieces and add them to the salad.

Fruity Curry Chicken Salad

Ingredients
- 4 skinless, boneless Chicken Pliers - cooked and diced
- 1 tsp celery, diced
- 4 green onions, sliced
- 1 Golden Delicious apple peeled, cored and diced
- 1/3 cup golden raisins
- 1/3 cup seedless green grapes, halved

- 1/2 cup sliced toasted pecans
- ⅛ teaspoon ground black pepper
- 1/2 tsp curry powder
- 3/4 cup light mayonnaise

Instructions
- Measure 1

A big bowl, combine the chicken, onion, celery, apple, celery, celery, pecans, pepper, curry powder, and carrot. Mix altogether. Drink!

Turmeric Chicken & Kale Salad With Honey Lime Dressing-Sirtfood Recipes

Notes: When planning beforehand, dress the salad 10 minutes before serving. The chicken might be substituted with beef chopped, sliced prawns, or fish. Vegetarians may use chopped mushrooms or cooked quinoa.

Ingredients

For your poultry

* 1 tsp ghee or 1 tablespoon coconut oil
* 1/2 moderate brown onion, diced
* 250 300 grams / 9 oz. Chicken mince or pops upward Chicken thighs
* 1 large garlic clove, finely-manicured
* 1 tsp turmeric powder
* 1teaspoon lime zest
* juice of 1/2 lime
* 1/2 tsp salt

For your salad
* 6 broccolini 2 or two cups of broccoli florets
* two tbsp pumpkin seeds (pepitas)
* 3 big kale leaves, stalks removed and sliced
* 1/2 avocado, chopped
* bunch of coriander leaves, chopped
* couple of fresh parsley leaves, chopped

For your dressing table
* 3 tbsp lime juice
* 1 small garlic clove, finely diced or grated
* 3 tbsp Extra-virgin Coconut Oil (I used 1. Tsp avocado oil and 2 tbsp EVO)
* 1 tsp raw honey
* 1/2 tsp Whole Grain or Dijon mustard
* 1/2 tsp sea salt and salt

Guidelines

1. Heat the ghee or coconut oil at a Tiny skillet Pan above medium-high heat. Bring the onion and then sauté on moderate heat for 45 minutes, until golden. Insert the chicken blossom and garlic and simmer for 2-3 minutes on medium-high heat, breaking it all out.

2. Add the garlic, lime zest, lime juice, and salt and Soda and cook stirring often, to get a further 3-4 minutes. Place the cooked mince aside.

3. As the chicken is cooking, make a little Spoonful of water. Insert the broccolini and cook 2 minutes. Rinse under warm water and then cut into 3-4 pieces each.

4. Insert the pumpkin seeds into the skillet out of the Toast and chicken over moderate heat for two minutes, stirring often to avoid burning. Season with a little salt. Setaside. Raw pumpkin seeds will also be nice to utilize.

5. Put chopped spinach at a salad bowl and then pour over The dressing table. With the hands, massage, and toss the carrot with the dressing table. This will dampen the lettuce, a lot similar to

what citrus juice will not steak or fish carpaccio – it 'hamburgers' it marginally.

6. Finally, throw throughout the cooked chicken, Broccolini, fresh herbs, pumpkin seeds, and avocado pieces.

Lamb, Butternut Squash And Date Tagine

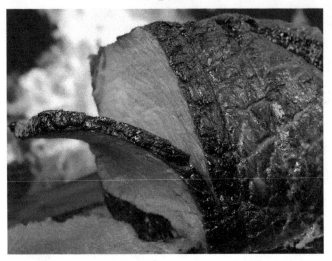

Incredible Warming Moroccan spices create this balanced tagine perfect for cold autumn and chilly evenings. Drink buckwheat to get an excess overall health kick!

Ingredients

2 Tsp coconut oil

1 Red onion, chopped

2cm ginger, grated

3 Garlic cloves, crushed or grated

1 teaspoon chili flakes (or to taste)

2 Tsp cumin seeds

1 cinnamon stick

2 teaspoons ground turmeric

800g lamb neck fillet, cut into 2cm chunks

1/2 Tsp salt

100g Medjool dates, pitted and sliced

400g Tin chopped berries, and half of a can of plain water

500g Butternut squash, chopped into 1cm cubes

400g Tin chickpeas, drained

2 Tsp fresh coriander (and extra for garnish)

Buckwheat, Cous-cous, flatbread or rice to function

Method

1. Pre Heat Your oven to 140C.

2. Drizzle Roughly 2 tbsp of coconut oil into a large ovenproof saucepan or cast-iron casserole dish. Add the chopped onion and cook on a gentle heat, with the lid for around five minutes, until the onions are softened but not too brown.

3. Insert The grated ginger and garlic, chili, cumin, cinnamon, and garlic. Stir well and cook 1 minute with off the lid. Add a dash of water when it becomes too humid.

4. Next, add from the lamb balls. Stir to coat the beef from the spices and onions, then add the salt chopped meats and berries and roughly half of a can of plain water (100-200ml).

5. Bring The tagine into the boil and put the lid and put on your skillet for about 1 hour and fifteen minutes.

6. Ten Moments prior to the conclusion of this cooking period, add the chopped butternut squash and drained chickpeas. Stir everything together, place the lid back and go back to the oven to the last half an hour of cooking.

7. When That, the tagine is able to remove from the oven and then stir fry throughout the chopped coriander. Drink buckwheat, couscous, flatbread, or basmati rice.

Notes

In case You really do not have an ovenproof saucepan or cast iron casserole dish, then only cook the tagine at a standard saucepan until it must go from the oven and transfer the tagine to a routine lidded skillet before placing in the oven. Add in an additional five minutes of cooking time and energy to allow the simple fact that the noodle dish will probably be needing additional time to warm up.

Prawn Arrabbiata-Sirtfood Recipes

Ingredients

125-150 G Beef or cooked prawns (Ideally king prawns)

65 Gram Buckwheat pasta

1 Tablespoon Extra virgin coconut oil

To get the arrabbiata sauce

40 G Red onion, finely chopped

1 Garlic clove, finely chopped

30 Gram celery, thinly sliced

1 Bird's eye chili, finely chopped

1 Tsp Dried mixed veggies

1 Tsp extra-virgin coconut oil

2 Tablespoon White wine (optional)

400 Gram Tinned chopped berries

1 tbsp Chopped parsley

Method

1. Fry the garlic, onion, celery, and peppermint and peppermint blossoms at the oil over moderate-low heat for 1--2 weeks. Turn up the heat to medium, bring the wine and cook 1 second. Add the berries and leave the sauce simmer over moderate-low heat for 20--half an hour, until it's a great rich texture. In the event you're feeling that the sauce is becoming too thick, simply put in just a very little water.

2. As the sauce is cooking, attract a bowl of water to the boil and then cook the pasta as per the package directions. Once cooked to

your dish, drain, then toss with the olive oil and also maintain at the pan before needed.

3. If you're utilizing raw prawns, put them into your sauce and cook for a further 3--four minutes, till they've turned opaque and pink, then add the parsley and function. If you're using cooked prawns, insert them using the skillet, then bring the sauce to the boil and then function.

4. Add the cooked pasta into the sauce, then mix thoroughly but lightly and function.

Turmeric Baked Salmon-Sirtfood Recipes
Ingredients
125-150 Gram Skinned Salmon
1 Tsp extra-virgin coconut oil
1 Tsp Ground turmeric
1/4 Juice of a lemon

To get The hot celery
1 Tsp extra-virgin coconut oil
40 G Red onion, finely chopped
60 Gram Tinned green peas
1 Garlic clove, finely chopped

1 Cm fresh ginger, finely chopped
1 Bird's eye chili, finely chopped
150 Gram Celery, cut into 2cm lengths
1 Tsp darkened curry powder
130 Gram Tomato, cut into 8 wedges
100 Ml vegetable or pasta stock
1 tbsp Chopped parsley

Method

Heat the oven to 200C / gas mark 6.

Start using the hot celery. Heat a skillet over moderate-low heat, then add the olive oil, then the garlic, onion, ginger, celery, and peppermint. Fry lightly for two-three minutes until softened but not colored, you can add the curry powder and cook for a further minute.

Insert the berries afterward, your lentils and stock, and simmer for 10 seconds. You might choose to increase or reduce the cooking time according to how crunchy you'd like your own sausage.

Meanwhile, mix the garlic olive oil and lemon juice and then rub the salmon. # Set on the baking dish and cook 8--10 seconds.

In order to complete, stir the skillet throughout the celery and function with the salmon.

Coronation Steak Salad-Sirtfood Recipes

Ingredients

75 G Natural yogurt

Juice Of 1/4 of a lemon

1 Tsp Coriander, sliced

1 Tsp Ground turmeric

1/2 Tsp darkened curry powder

100 G Cooked chicken, cut to bite-sized pieces

6 Walnut halves, finely chopped

1 Medjool date, finely chopped

20 G Crimson pumpkin, diced

1 Bird's eye illuminates

40 Gram Rocket, to function

Method

Mix The lemon, carrot juice, spices, and coriander together in a bowl. Add all of the remaining ingredients and serve on a bed of this rocket.

Baked Potatoes With Spicy Chickpea Stew-Sirtfood Recipes

Kind Of Mexican fauna matches North African Taginethis Spicy Chickpea Stew is very flavorful and also makes an excellent topping for baked potatoes, also it simply appears to be vegan, vegetarian, gluten-free and dairy-free. Plus, it comprises chocolate.

Ingredients

4 6 Celery, pricked all over

2 Tsp coconut oil

2 Red onions, finely chopped

4 Cloves garlic, crushed or grated

2cm ginger, grated

1/2 -2 teaspoons chili flakes (depending on how hot you enjoy stuff)

2 tablespoons cumin seeds

2 Tsp turmeric

Splash Of water

2 x 400g tins chopped tomatoes

2 Tablespoons unsweetened cocoa powder (or even cacao)

2 X 400g tins chickpeas (or kidney beans if you would like) including the chick-pea water do not DRAIN!!

2 Yellow peppers (or any color you would like!) , chopped into bitesize pieces

2 Tablespoons parsley and extra for garnish

Salt And pepper to taste

Negative Salad

Method

1. Pre Heat The oven to 200C, however, you are able to prepare all of your own ingredients.

2. When The oven is still hot enough to set your lemon potatoes from the oven and cook for 1 hour or so until they do the way you prefer them.

3. Once The potatoes come from the oven, then place the coconut oil and sliced red onion into a large wide saucepan and cook lightly, with the lid for five minutes until the onions are tender but not brown.

4. Remove The lid and then add the ginger, garlic, cumin, and simmer. Cook for a further minute on very low heat, then add the garlic and a tiny dab of water and then cook for another moment, just take care never to allow the pan to get too tender.

5. Next, Add from the berries, cocoa powder (or even cacao), chickpeas (including the chickpea water) and salt. Bring to the boil, and then simmer on a very low heat for 4-5 seconds before the sauce is thick and unctuous (but do not allow it to burn up) .

The stew ought to be performed at exactly the exact same period as the legumes.

6. Finally, Stir at the two tbsp of parsley, plus a few pepper and salt if you desire, and also serve the stew in addition to the chopped sausage, possibly with a very simple salad.

Kale And Red Onion Dhal With Buckwheat-Sirtfood Recipes

Delicious And very wholesome, this Kale and Red Onion Dhal using Buckwheat are quick and simple to generate and naturally gluten-free, dairy-free, vegetarian, and vegetarian.

INGREDIENTS
1 Tbsp coconut oil
1 Small red onion, chopped
3 Garlic cloves, crushed or grated
2 Cm lemon, grated
1 Birdseye chili, deseeded and finely chopped (more if you like things sexy!)
2 Tsp turmeric
2 teaspoons garam masala
160g Red lentils
400ml Coconut milk
200ml Water

100g Kale (or lettuce are a terrific alternative)

160g buckwheat (or brown rice)

METHOD

1. Put The coconut oil in a large, deep saucepan and then add the chopped onion. Cook on very low heat, with the lid for five minutes until softened.

2. Insert The ginger, garlic, and chili and cook 1 minute.

3. Insert The garlic, garam masala, and a dash of water and then cook for 1 minute.

4. Insert The reddish peas, coconut milk, and also 200ml water (try so only by half filling the coconut milk could with water and stirring it in the saucepan).

5. Mix Everything together thoroughly and then cook for 20 minutes over a lightly heat with the lid . Stir occasionally and add just a little bit more water in case the dhal starts to stand.

6. Later 20 seconds add the carrot, stir thoroughly and then replace the lid, then cook for a further five minutes (1 2 minutes if you are using spinach)

7. Around 1-5 minutes ahead of the curry is ready, set the buckwheat at a medium saucepan, and then put in lots of warm water. Bring back the water to the boil and then cook for 10 minutes (or only a little longer in case you would rather your buckwheat softer. Drain the buckwheat at a sieve and function with the dhal.

Char-grilled Steak Having A Dark Wine Jus, Onion Rings, Garlic Kale, And Herb Roasted Potatoes

INGREDIENTS:

100g potatoes, peeled and cut into 2cm dice

1 Tbsp extra virgin coconut oil

5g parsley, finely chopped

50g Red onion, chopped into circles

50g Lettuce, chopped

1 garlic clove, finely chopped

120--150g X-ray 3.5cm-thick beef noodle beef or 2cm-thick sirloin beef

40ml Red wine

150ml Beef inventory
1 Tsp tomato purée
1 Tsp cornflour, dissolved in 1 tablespoon water

Guidelines:

Heating The oven to 220°C/gas .

Put The sausage in a saucepan of boiling water, then return to the boil and then cook 4minutes, then empty. Put in a skillet with 1 tbsp of the oil and then roast in the oven for 3-5 --4-5 minutes. Twist the berries every 10 minutes to ensure even cooking. After cooked remove from the oven, sprinkle with the chopped parsley and mix well.

Fry The onion 1 tsp of the oil over a moderate heat for 5 minutes - 1 minute, until tender and well caramelized. Maintain heat. Steam the kale for two-three minutes . Stir the garlic lightly in 1/2 tsp of oil for 1 minute, until tender but not colored. Insert the spinach and simmer for a further 1--two minutes, until tender. Maintain heat.

Heating An ovenproof skillet on high heat until smoking. Lay the beef from 1/2 a tsp of the oil and then fry from the skillet over a moderate-highgh temperature in accordance with just how you would like your beef done.If you prefer your beef moderate, it'd be wise to sear the beef and also transfer the pan into a toaster place in 220°C/petrol 7 and then finish the cooking which manner to your prescribed occasions.

Remove The meat from the pan and put aside to break. Add your wine into the skillet to bring any meat up residue. Bubble to decrease the wine by half an hour until syrupy, along with a flavor that is concentrated.

Insert The inventory and tomato purée into the beef pan and bring to the boil, add the cornflour paste to thicken your sauce, then adding it only a little at a time till you've got your preferred consistency. Stir in just about anyone of those juices out of the dinner that is rested and serve with the roasted lettuce, celery, onion rings, and red berry sauce.

Kale And Black-currant Smoothie

2 Tsp honey
1 Cup freshly made green-tea
10 Infant spinach leaves stalk removed
1 Ripe banana
40 Gram blackcurrants washed and stalk removed
6 Ice cubes

Stir The honey to the green tea before dissolved. Whiz each of the ingredients together in a blender until smooth. Drink instantly.

DINNER RECIPES

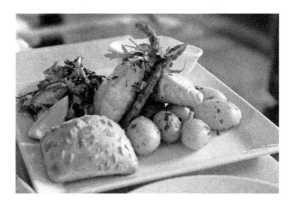

Pesto salmon pasta noodles recipe

Ingredients

- 350g penne
- 2 x 212g tins cherry salmon, drained
- 1 lemon, zested and juiced
- 190g jar green pesto
- 250g package cherry tomatoes halved
- 100g bunch spring onions, finely chopped
- 125g package reduced-fat mozzarella

Method

1. Preheat the oven to Windows 7, 220°C, buff 200°C. Boil the pasta for 5 mins. Drain, reserving 100ml drinking water.
2. Meanwhile, at a 2ltr ovenproof dish, then mix the salmon, lemon zest, and juice, then pesto (booking 2 tablespoons)berries and half of the spring onions; season.
3. Mix the pasta and reserved cooking water to the dish. Mix the allowed pesto using 1 tablespoon water and then drizzle on the pasta. Gently within the mozzarella, top with the rest of the spring onions and bake for 25 mins until golden.

Sri Lankan-style sweet potato curry recipe

Ingredients

- 1/2 onion, roughly sliced
- 3 garlic cloves, roughly sliced
- 25g sliced ginger, chopped and peeled
- 15g fresh coriander stalks and leaves split leaves sliced
- two 1/2 tablespoon moderate tikka curry powder
- 60g package cashew nuts
- 1 tablespoon olive oil
- 500g Redmere Farms sweet potatoes, peeled and cut into 3cm balls

- 400ml tin Isle Sun Coconut-milk
- 1/2 vegetable stock block, created as much as 300ml
- 200g Grower's Harvest long-grain rice
- 300g frozen green beans
- 150g Redmere Farms lettuce
- 1 Suntrail Farms lemon, 1/2 juiced, 1/2 cut into wedges to function

Method

1. Set the onion, ginger, garlic, coriander stalks, tikka powder along with half of the cashew nuts in a food processor. Insert 2 tablespoons water and blitz to a chunky paste.
2. At a large skillet, warm the oil over moderate heat. Insert the paste and cook, stirring for 5 mins. Bring the sweet potatoes, stir, then pour into the coconut milk and stock. Bring to the simmer and boil for 25-35 mins before the sweet potatoes are tender.
3. Meanwhile, cook the rice pack directions. Toast the rest of the cashews at a dry skillet.
4. Sti-R the beans into the curry and then simmer for two mins. Insert the lettuce in handfuls, allowing each to simmer before adding the following; simmer for 1 minute. Bring the lemon juice, to taste, & the majority of the

coriander leaves. Scatter on the remaining coriander and cashews, then use the rice and lemon wedges.

Chicken liver along with tomato ragu recipe

Ingredients

- 2 tablespoon olive oil
- 1 onion, finely chopped
- 2 carrots, scrubbed and simmer
- 4 garlic cloves, finely chopped
- 1/4 x 30g pack fresh ginger, stalks finely chopped, leaves ripped
- 380g package poultry livers, finely chopped, and almost any sinew removed and lost
- 400g tin Grower's Harvest chopped berries
- 1 chicken stock cube, created around 300ml
- 1/2 tsp caster sugar
- 300g penne
- 1/4 Suntrail Farms lemon, juiced

Method

1. Heat 1 tablespoon oil in a large skillet, over a low-medium heating system. Fry the onion and carrots to 10 mins,

stirring periodically. Stir in the ginger and garlic pops and cook 2 mins more. Transfer into a bowl set aside.
2. Twist the pan into high heat and then add the oil. Bring the chicken livers and simmer for 5 mins until browned. Pour the onion mix to the pan and then stir in the tomatoes, sugar, and stock. Season, bring to the boil, and then simmer for 20 mins until reduced and thickened, and also the liver is cooked through. Meanwhile, cook pasta to package guidelines.
3. Taste the ragu and put in a second pinch of sugar more seasoning, if needed. Put in a squeeze of lemon juice to taste and stir in two of the ripped basil leaves. Divide the pasta between four bowls, then spoon across the ragu and top with the rest of the basil.

Minted Lamb with a couscous salad recipe
Ingredients

- 75g Cous-cous
- 1/2 chicken stock block, composed to 125ml
- 30g pack refreshing flat-leaf parsley, sliced
- 3 mint sprigs, leaves picked and sliced
- 1 tablespoon olive oil

- 200g pack suspended BBQ minted lamb leg beans, Defrosted
- 200g lettuce berries, sliced
- 1/4 tsp, sliced
- 1 spring onion, sliced
- pinch of ground cumin
- 1/2 lemon, zested and juiced
- 50g reduced-fat salad cheese

Method

1. Place the couscous into a heatproof bowl and then pour on the inventory. Cover and set aside for 10 mins, then fluff with a fork and stir in the herbs.
2. Meanwhile, rub a little oil within the lamb steaks and season. Cook to package guidelines, then slit.
3. Mix the tomatoes, cucumber and spring onion into the couscous with the oil, the cumin, and lemon juice and zest. Crumble on the salad and serve with the bunny.

Jack Fruit tortilla bowls recipe

To get A winning beef - and - dairy-free dinner idea for just two, look no farther than this particular colorful Mexican Jack fruit recipe. With barbecued legumes, corn, and brilliant veg, you are going to wish to create this simple vegetarian meal over and over. See strategy

- Serves 2
- 5 mins to prepare and 15 mins to cook
- 354 calories serving
- healthful

Ingredients

- Two Sweet Corn cobettes
- 1 red chili, finely chopped
- 2 teaspoon olive oil
- 1 lime, juiced
- 15g fresh coriander, chopped, plus extra to garnish
- 150g package stained Jack Fruit in Texmex sauce
- 210g tin kidney beans, drained
- 125g roasted red peppers (in the jar), drained and chopped
- two whitened tortilla packs
- 1/2 round lettuce, ripped

Method

- Heat a griddle Pan on a high temperature (or light a barbecue). Griddle that the cobettes to get 10 12 Mins, turning until cooked and charred throughout. Remove from the pan and also Stand upright onto a plank. Use a sharp knife to carefully reduce the Span of this corn, staying near to the heart, to clear away the kernels. Mix That the kernels with the eucalyptus oil, half of the carrot juice along with half an hour of the coriander.
- Heating the Jack fruit and sauce in a saucepan with the legumes, peppers, staying lime Coriander and juice on medium-low heating for 3-4 mins until heated Through; now.

Griddle the wraps for 10 20 secs each side to char. Tear into pieces and serve together with all the Jack Fruit lettuce And sweet corn salsa.

Carrot, courgette and halloumi Hamburgers recipe
Want Some veggie beans inspiration for the next grill? This carrot, courgette, and halloumi hamburger recipe is packaged with grated veg and creates a switch from bean hamburgers. Layer up using chopped tzatziki, delicate pineapple ribbons, and salad for a simple vegetarian barbecue winner. See strategy

- Serves 4

- 20 mins to prepare and 10 mins to cook
- 523 calories serving
- wholesome

Ingredients

- 1 big carrot, grated
- 1 large courgette, grated
- 225g halloumi, grated
- 2 spring onions, finely chopped
- 90g Bread Crumbs
- 1 tablespoon ground cumin
- 1 tablespoon ground coriander
- 1/2 teaspoon salt
- 2 tbsp
- Two tablespoons flour
- 4 brioche buns, halved
- 50g baby spinach leaves
- 1 big tomato, sliced
- 1 small red onion, chopped
- 1/2 pineapple, peeled into ribbons
- tzatziki, to function

Method

1. Place the courgette into a clean tea towel and squeeze to eradicate any liquid. Hint into a big bowl and then add the carrot, halloumi, onion, bread crumbs, cumin, coriander, eggs, salt, and flour. Stir well to mix.
2. Put simply over half the mix in a food processor and pulse until the mixture starts to stay . Reunite back this into the booked mix and mix well.
3. Divide the mix into 4 and then form into patties. Heat a grill or griddle pan into a moderate heat. Cook the hamburgers for 45 mins each side until golden and cooked through.
4. Insert the hamburger buns into the grill till lightly toasted. To assemble the burgers, put lettuce leaves on the base of each bun. Top with all the hamburger, a piece of tomato, pineapple ribbon along with a spoonful of tzatziki.

Rita's 'Rowdy' enchiladas recipe

When They all remain, Rita's kiddies really are a rowdy group. But there is something that is sure to create a silent silence into the dining table, which is her chicken enchiladas. Made out of sweet red peppers, Chicken feeding, and spices wrapped up within tortilla wraps and roasted with a spicy black bean tomato sauce and grated cheese, then it is not Tough to see exactly why. View method

- Serves 4
- 1-5 mins to prepare and 55 mins to cook
- 757 carbs serving
- Freezable

Ingredients

- Two large chicken breasts (about 400g)
- 2 red peppers, thinly chopped
- 1 tablespoon olive oil
- 3/4 tsp mild chili powder
- 1 teaspoon 1/2 tsp ground cumin
- 3/4 tsp smoked paprika
- 80g grated mozzarella
- 8 Plain Tortilla Wraps
- 65g ripe Cheddar, grated
- 10g fresh coriander, roughly sliced

The sauce

- 1 tablespoon olive oil
- 1/2 onion, finely chopped
- 2 tsp cloves, crushed
- 500g tomato passata

- 1 tablespoon chipotle chili paste
- 400g tin black beans drained and rinsed
- 1/2 lime, juiced

Method

1. Preheat the oven to gas 5, 190°C, buff 170°C. Set the chicken at a 20 x 30cm skillet with all the pepper olive oil, chili powder, cumin, and paprika. Mix to coat, then cover with foil. Roast for 25-30 mins before the chicken is cooked and tender with no pink meat remains. Take out the chicken from the dish and then shred with two forks. Reserve in a bowl.
2. Meanwhile, make the sauce. Heat the oil in a saucepan on a low heat and cook the garlic and onion for 10 mins. Stir from the passata and chipotle chili glue; increase heat to moderate, bring to a simmer and cook for a further 10 mins, stirring periodically. Bring the beans and carrot juice season.
3. Mix one-third of this sauce plus half of the mozzarella to the cultured broccoli and chicken.
4. To gather, spoon 4 tablespoons of this sauce in exactly the exact baking dish before. Spoon a bit of the chicken mixture down the middle of each tortilla, roll up, and then put it from the dish. Repeat with the tortillas and filling, then placing them alongside in order that they do not

shatter. Pour the remaining sauce on the top and then scatter within the Cheddar and remaining mozzarella. Bake in the oven for 20-25 mins until the cheese has melted and begun to brownish. Scatter together with all the coriander to function.

Freezing And defrosting recommendations

Cook As educated and let it cool completely. Subsequently, move to an airtight, freezer-safe container, seal, and freeze up to 1-3 weeks. Guarantee the meatballs are underwater in the sauce since they are going to freeze far better. To serve, defrost thoroughly in the refrigerator overnight before reheating. To serve, put in a bowl over moderate heat, stirring occasionally until the dish is heated throughout.

Full-of-veg hash recipe

To get A simple solution to lure all of the households to eat more veg, try out this curry hash recipe together with carrots, onions, courgettes, parsley, and topped with an egg. This family preferred is created from massaging the veg, meaning there is hardly any hands-free moment; therefore, it's fantastic for rapping through to busy weeknights. See strategy

Ingredients

- 750g potatoes, pared and grated
- 2 tablespoon olive oil
- 100g streaky bacon, roughly sliced
- 2 red onions, finely chopped
- 300g carrots, peeled and diced
- two courgettes, diced
- 2 garlic cloves, crushed
- 4 eggs
- 5g refreshing flat-leaf parsley, sliced
- 1 red chili, chopped (optional)
- 1/2 x 340g jar pickled red cabbage

Method

1. Preheat the oven to Windows 7, 220°C, buff 200°C. Bring a bowl of soapy water to the boil and then simmer the potatoes for 5 mins, then drain and put aside.
2. Heat 1 tablespoon oil in a large, ovenproof skillet on a high heat and fry the bacon for 5 mins until crispy. Add the carrots, onions, courgettes, onions, and garlic; season and then cook for 5 mins. Transfer the pan into the oven and bake for 25-30 mins before the veg is tender and gold.

3. Meanwhile, heat the remaining oil into a skillet on medium-high heating and fry the eggs 2-3 mins or until cooked to your liking.
4. Split the hash between two plates and top each with lettuce. Scatter with parsley and simmer, then function with the pickled red cabbage onto both

Bacon and egg fried rice recipe

Cook This up egg and bacon fried rice for a fast and effortless d,inner. Adding streaky bacon brings extra feel and flavor for the wallet-friendly stirfry. See strategy

Ingredients

- 350g long-grain rice, well rinsed
- 1 1/2 tablespoon olive oil
- 100g streaky bacon, diced
- two peppers, finely chopped
- 2 red onions, finely chopped
- 200g carrots, peeled and coarsely grated
- 2 garlic cloves, crushed
- 5cm slice ginger, peeled and grated
- 1 red chili, finely chopped (optional)

- 2 eggs
- 2 tsp soy sauce

Method

- Cook the rice in a big bowl of warm water for 10 mins until not quite tender. Drain, rinse with warm water and drain . Setaside.
- Meanwhile, warm 1/2 tablespoon oil in a skillet on a high heat and fry the bacon for 5 7 mins until golden and crispy. Remove from the pan using a slotted spoon and place aside. Add 1 tablespoon oil and fry the peppers for 10 mins until lightly bubbling. Add the carrots, onions, ginger, garlic, and chili and fry over a moderate-high temperature for 5 mins more.
- Insert the rice and bacon and simmer for 5 mins, stirring often. Push the rice mix to a single side of this pan and then crack the eggs to the gap. Beat the eggs with a wooden spoon, then stir throughout the rice. Cook for 2 mins, then add the soy sauce and then remove from heat. Split between 4 shallow bowls to function.

Super-speedy prawn risotto

Heating 1 tablespoon coconut oil in a skillet on medium-high heat and then put in 100g Diced Onion; cook 5 mins. Insert 2 x 250g packs whole-grain Rice & Quinoa along with 175ml hot vegetable stock (or plain water), together side 200g suspended Garden Peas. Gently split using rice using a wooden spoon. Cover and cook 3 mins, stirring occasionally, you can add two x 150g packs Cooked and Peeled King Prawns. Cook for 12 mins before prawns, peas, and rice have been piping hot, and the majority of the liquid was consumed. Remove from heat. Chop 1/2 x 85g tote water-cress and stir throughout; up to taste. Top with watercress leaves and pepper to function.

Ingredients:

100g Diced Onion

Two X 250g packs whole-grain Rice & Quinoa

200g Frozen Garden Peas

Two x 150g packs Cooked and Peeled King Prawns

1/285g Tote water-cress

SNACKS & DESSERTS RECIPES

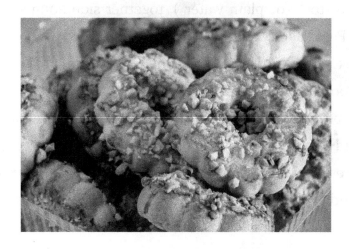

Lemon Ricotta Cookies with Lemon Glaze

Ingredients

- Two 1/2 cups all-purpose flour
- 1 tsp baking powder
- 1 tsp salt
- 1 tbsp unsalted butter softened
- 2 cups of sugar
- 2 capsules
- 1 teaspoon (15-ounce) container whole-milk ricotta cheese
- 3 tbsp lemon juice
- 1 lemon, zested

- Glaze:
- 1 1/2 cups powdered sugar
- 3 tbsp lemon juice
- 1 lemon, zested

Guidelines

1. Preheat the oven to 375 degrees F.
2. At a medium bowl, combine the flour, baking powder, and salt. Setaside.
3. From the big bowl, blend the butter and the sugar levels. With an electric mixer, beat the sugar and butter until light and fluffy, about three minutes. Add the eggs1 at a time, beating until incorporated.
4. Insert the ricotta cheese, lemon juice, and lemon zest. Beat to blend. Stir in the dry skin.
5. Line two baking sheets with parchment paper. Spoon the dough (approximately 2 tablespoons of each cookie) on the baking sheets. Bake for fifteen minutes, until slightly golden at the borders. Remove from the oven and allow the biscuits remaining baking sheet for about 20 minutes.
6. Glaze:
7. Combine the powdered sugar lemon juice and lemon peel in a small bowl and then stir until smooth. Spoon approximately 1/2-tsp on each cookie and make use of the back of the spoon to lightly disperse. Allow glaze harden

for approximately two hours. Pack the biscuits to a decorative jar.

Home-made Marshmallow Fluff

Ingredients

- 3/4 cup sugar
- 1/2 cup light corn syrup
- 1/4 cup water
- ⅛ tsp salt
- 3 little egg whites egg whites
- 1/4 tsp cream of tartar
- 1 teaspoon 1/2 tsp vanilla infusion

Guidelines

1. In a little pan, mix together sugar, corn syrup, salt, and water. Attach a candy thermometer into the side of this pan, which makes sure it will not touch the underside of the pan. Setaside.
2. From the bowl of a stand mixer, combine egg whites and cream of tartar. Begin to whip on medium speed with the whisk attachment.

3. Meanwhile, turn the burner on top and place the pan with the sugar mix onto heat. Allow mix into a boil and heat to 240 degrees, stirring periodically.
4. The aim is to find the egg whites whipped to soft peaks and also the sugar heated to 240 degrees at near the same moment. Simply stop stirring the egg whites once they hit soft peaks.
5. Once the sugar has already reached 240 amounts, turn noodle onto reducing. Insert a little quantity of the popular sugar mix and let it mix. Insert still another little sum of the sugar mix. Carry on to add mix slowly, and that means you never scramble the egg whites.
6. After all of the sugar was added into the egg whites, then turn the rate of this mixer and also keep to overcome concoction for around 79 minutes until the fluff remains glossy and stiff. In roughly the 5 minute mark, then add vanilla extract.
7. Use fluff immediately or store in an airtight container in the fridge for around two weeks.

Guilt Totally free Banana Icecream
Ingredients

- 3 quite ripe banana - peeled and rooted
- a couple of chocolate chips

- two Tbsp skim milk

Guidelines

1. Throw all ingredients into a food processor and blend until creamy.
2. Eat freeze and appreciate afterward.

Perfect Little PB Snack Balls

Ingredients

- 1/2 cup chunky peanut butter
- 3 Tbsp flax seeds
- 3 Tbsp wheat germ
- 1 Tbsp honey or agave
- 1/4 cup powder

Guidelines

1. Blend dry ingredients and adding from the honey and peanut butter.
2. Mix well and roll into chunks and then conclude by rolling into wheatgerm.

Dark Chocolate Pretzel Cookies

Ingredients

- 1 cup yogurt
- 1/2 tsp baking soda
- 1/4 teaspoon salt
- 1/4 tsp cinnamon
- 4 Tbsp butter softened
- 1/3 cup brown sugar
- 1 egg
- 1/2 tsp vanilla
- 1/2 cup dark chocolate chips
- 1/2 cup pretzelstsp chopped

Guidelines

1. Pre Heat oven to 350 degrees.
2. At a medium bowl, whisk together the sugar, butter, vanilla, and egg.
3. In another bowl, stir together the flour, baking soda, and salt.

4. Stir the bread mixture in using all the moist components, along with the chocolate chips and pretzels until just blended.
5. Drop large spoonfuls of dough on an unlined baking sheet.
6. Bake for 15-17 minutes, or until the bottoms are somewhat all crispy.
7. Allow cooling on a wire rack.

Mascarpone Cheesecake with Almond Crust
Ingredients

- Crust
- 1/2 cup slivered almonds
- 8 tsp -- or 2/3 cup graham cracker crumbs
- 2 tbsp sugar
- 1 tbsp salted butter melted
- Filling
- 1 (8-ounce) packages cream cheese, room temperature
- 1 (8-ounce) container mascarpone cheese, room temperature
- 3/4 cup sugar
- 1 tsp fresh lemon juice (I needed to use imitation Lemon-juice)
- 1 tsp vanilla infusion
- 2 large eggs, room temperature

Guidelines

1. For the crust: Preheat oven to 350 degrees F.Take per 9-inch diameter around the pan (I had a throw off). Finely grind the almonds, cracker crumbs sugar in a food processor or (I used my magic bullet). Bring the butter and process until moist crumbs form.
2. Press the almond mixture on the base of the prepared pan (maybe not on the surfaces of the pan). Bake the crust until it's put and start to brown, about 1-2 minutes. Cool. Decrease the oven temperature to 325 degrees F.
3. for your filling: With an electric mixer, beat the cream cheese, mascarpone cheese, and sugar in a large bowl until smooth, occasionally scraping down the sides of the jar using a rubber spatula. Beat in the lemon juice and vanilla. Add the eggs1 at a time, beating until combined after each addition.
4. Pour the cheese mixture on the crust from the pan. Put the pan into a big skillet or Pyrex dish Pour enough hot water to the roasting pan to come halfway up ,the sides of one's skillet. Bake until the middle of this racket goes slightly when the pan is gently shaken, about 1 hour (the dessert will get business if it's cold). Transfer the cake to a stand; trendy for 1 hour. Refrigerate before the cheesecake is cold, at least eight hours.

5. ToppingI squeezed just a small thick cream at the microwave using a busted up Lindt chocolate brown -- afterward, the got a Ziploc baggie and cut out a hole at the corner then poured the melted chocolate to the baggie and used this to decorate the cake!

Marshmallow Pop Corn Balls

Ingredients

- 2 bag of microwave popcorn
- 1 12.6 ounces. Tote M&M's
- 3 cups honey roasted peanuts
- 1 pkg. 16 ounce. Massive marshmallows
- 1 cup butter, cubed

Guidelines

1. In a bowl, blend the popcorn, peanuts and M&M's.
2. In a big pot, combine marshmallows and butter.
3. Cook medium-low warmth .
4. Insert popcorn mix, blend nicely
5. Spray muffin tins with nonstop cooking spray.

6. When cool enough to handle, spray hands together with nonstick cooking spray and then shape into chunks and put into a muffin tin to carry contour.
7. Add popsicle stick into each chunk and then let cool.
8. Wrap each person in vinyl when chilled.

Home-made Ice-cream Drumsticks
Ingredients

- Vanilla ice cream
- Two Lindt Hazel Nut chunks
- magical shell - out chocolate
- sugar levels
- nuts (I mixed crushed peppers and unsalted peanuts)
- parchment newspaper

Guidelines
- Soften ice cream and mixin topping - I had two sliced Lindt hazel nutballs.
- Fill underside of sugar with magic and nuts shell and top with ice cream.
- Wrap parchment paper round cone and then fill cone over about 1.5 inches across the cap of the cone (the newspaper can help to carry its shape).

- Shirt with magical nuts and shells.
- Freeze for about 20 minutes before the ice cream is business.

Ultimate Chocolate Chip Cookie n' Oreo Fudge Brownie Bar

Ingredients

- 1 cup (2 sticks) butter, softened
- 1 cup granulated sugar
- 3/4 cup light brown sugar
- two big egg
- 1 Tablespoon pure vanilla extract
- two 1/2 cups all-purpose flour
- 1 tsp baking soda
- 1 tsp lemon
- 2 cups (12 oz) milk chocolate chips
- 1 pkg Double Stuffed Oreos
- 1 Family-size (9×13) Brownie mixture
- 1/4 cup hot fudge topping

Guidelines

1. Pre Heat oven to 350 degrees F.
2. Cream the butter and sugars in a large bowl using an electric mixer at medium speed for 35 minutes.
3. Add the vanilla and eggs and mix well to thoroughly combine. In another bowl, whisk together the flour,

baking soda and salt, and slowly incorporate in the mixer till the bread is simply combined.
4. Stir in chocolate chips.
5. Spread the cookie dough at the bottom of a 9×1-3 baking dish that is wrapped with wax nonstick then coated with cooking spray.
6. cloth with a coating of Oreos. Mix together brownie mix, adding an optional 1/4 cup of hot fudge directly into the mixture.
7. Twist the brownie batter within the Cookie-dough and Oreos.
8. Cover with foil and bake at 350 degrees F for half an hour.
9. Remove foil and continue baking for another 15 25 minutes.
10. Let cool before cutting on brownies might nevertheless be gooey at the midst while warm, but will also place up perfectly once chilled.

Crunchy Chocolate Chip Coconut Macadamia Nut Cookies

Ingredients

- 1 cup yogurt
- 1/2 tsp baking soda
- 1/2 tsp salt

- 1 tbsp of butter, softened
- 1 cup firmly packed brown sugar
- 1/2 cup sugar
- 1 big egg
- 1/2 cup Semi-Sweet chocolate chips
- 1/2 cup sweetened flaked coconut
- 1/2 cup coarsely chopped dry-roasted the macadamia nuts
- 1/2 cup craisins

Guidelines

1. Preheat the oven to 325°F.
2. In a little bowl, whisk together the flour, oats and baking soda, and salt then places aside.
3. On your mixer bowl, then mix together the butter/sugar/egg mix.
4. Mix from the flour/oats mix until just combined and stir into the chocolate chips, craisins, nuts, and coconut.
5. Decked outsized bits on a parchment-lined cookie sheet.
6. Bake for 1-3 minutes before biscuits are only barely golden brown.
7. Remove from the oven and then leave the cookie sheets to cool at least 10 minutes.

Peach and Blueberry Pie

Ingredients

- Peach and Blueberry Pie
- Ingredients1 box of noodle dough
- Filling
- 5 peaches, peeled and chopped - that I used roasted peaches
- 3 cups strawberries
- 3/4 cup sugar
- 1/4 cup bread
- juice of 1/2 lemon
- 1 egg yolk, crushed

Guidelines

1. Pre Heat oven to 400 degrees.
2. Blend dough to a 9-inch pie plate.
3. In a big bowl, combine tomatoes, sugar, bread, and lemon juice, then toss to combine. Pour into the pie plate, mounding at the center.
4. Simply take an instant disk of bread and then cut into bits, then put a pie shirt and put the dough in addition to pressing on edges .

5. Brush crust with egg wash then sprinkles with sugar.
6. Set onto a parchment paper-lined baking sheet.
7. Bake at 400 for about 20 minutes, until crust is browned at borders.
8. Turn oven down to 350, bake for another 40 minutes.
9. Remove and let sit at least 30minutes.
10. Drink Vanilla Icecream.

Pear, Cranberry and Chocolate Crisp
Ingredients

- Crumble Topping:
- 1/2 cup pasta
- 1/2 cup brown sugar
- 1 tsp cinnamon
- 1/8 tsp salt
- 3/4 cup yogurt
- 1/4 cup sliced peppers
- 1/3 cup butter, melted
- 1 teaspoon vanilla
- tsp:
- 1 tbsp brown sugar
- 3 tsp, cut into balls
- 1/4 cup dried cranberries

- 1 teaspoon lemon juice
- two handfuls of milk chocolate chips

Guidelines

1. Pre Heat oven to 375.
2. Spray a casserole dish with a butter spray.
3. Put all of the topping ingredients - flour, sugar, cinnamon, salt, nuts, legumes, and dried
4. butter into a bowl and then mix. Setaside.
5. In a large bowl, combine the sugar, lemon juice, pears, and cranberries.
6. Once fully blended, move to the prepared baking dish.
7. Spread the topping evenly over the fruit.
8. Stinks for about half an hour.
9. Eliminate oven stir up - disperse chocolate chips out at the top.
10. Cook for another 10 minutes.
11. Drink ice cream.

Apricot Oatmeal Cookies

Ingredients

- 1/2 cup (1 stick) butter, softened
- 2/3 cup light brown sugar packed

- 1 egg
- 3/4 cup all-purpose flour
- 1/2 tsp baking soda
- 1/2 tsp vanilla infusion
- 1/2 tsp cinnamon
- 1/4 tsp salt
- 1 teaspoon 1/2 cups chopped oats
- 3/4 cup yolks
- 1/4 cup sliced apricots
- 1/3 cup slivered almonds

Guidelines

1. Preheat oven to 350°.
2. In a big bowl, combine with the butter, sugar, and egg until smooth.
3. In another bowl, whisk the flour, baking soda, cinnamon, and salt together.
4. Stir the dry ingredients to the butter-sugar bowl.
5. Now stir in the oats, raisins, apricots, and almonds.
6. I heard on the web that in this time -- it's much better to cool with the dough (therefore your biscuits are thicker)
7. Afterward, I scooped my biscuits into some parchment-lined (easier removal and wash up) cookie sheet - around two inches apart.

8. I sliced mine for approximately ten minutes - that they were fantastic!

21 DAY MEAL-PLAN

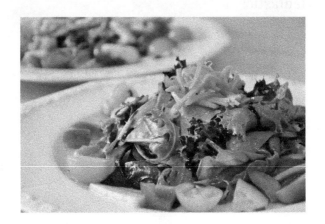

Day 1

Breakfast:

Cranberry Pecan Overnight Oats

Snack: Cucumber pieces with hummus

Lunch:

Avocado Tuna Salad or Shredded Tofu Pesto Sandwich

Snack: Apple pieces sprinkled with cinnamon and almonds

Dinner:

Left Overs: Turkey, Kale and Cauliflower Soup or Navy Bean Soup with Crispy Kale

Day 2
Breakfast:

Grain-Free Pumpkinseed Breakfast Cereal

Snack: Pear and almonds

Lunch:
Left Overs: Hearty Bean Chowder

Snack: Corn Thin Cakes with Guacamole and Fresh Salsa

Dinner:

Orange Chicken using Simple Salad OR Orange To-Fu

Day 3

Breakfast:

Sterile Eating Egg and Vegetable Basil Scramble OR Cheesy Tofu Scramble

Snack: Celery sticks with peanut butter and raisins

Lunch:

Left-over Taco Salad or Wild Rice Burrito Bowl

Snack: Orange and also a Hard-boiled egg or couple of roasted chickpeas

Dinner:

Turkey, Kale along with Cauliflower Soup or Navy Bean Soup with Crispy Kale

Day 4
Breakfast:

Morning Meal Egg Muffins OR Chickpea Flour Omelet Muffins OR sterile Eating Peanut Buttercup Oatmeal

Snack: Banana slices with peanut butter

Lunch:

Fiesta Chicken Salad Or Easy Broccoli Salad with Almond Lemon Dressing

Snack:1/2 Cucumber with two tbsp hummus

Dinner:

Garlic Shrimp in Coconut Coffee, Tomatoes and CilantroOR Zucchini, Pea and Spinach Pesto Risotto

Day 5

Breakfast:
Protein PancakesOR Paleo Vegan Pancakes

Snack: Pear and pistachios

Lunch:

Orange Almond Salad using Avocadoor Fall Harvest Salad with Pomegranate VinaigretteSnack: Skinny Pop popcorn along with Hard-Boiled egg

Dinner:

Seafood Zucchini Pasta OR Avocado Pesto Zucchini Noodles

Day 6

Breakfast:

Left Overs: Re Heated Protein or Vegan Pancakes

Snack: Banana slices with peanut butter

Lunch:
Left Overs: Seafood Zucchini Pasta or Avocado Pesto Zucchini Noodles

Snack: Baby carrots along with guacamole

Dinner:

Sterile Eating Hearty Bean Chowder

Day 7
Breakfast:

Left-over Egg or Chick-pea Muffins OR sterile Eating Peanut Buttercup Oatmeal

Snack: Apple with Sun-flower seed/pumpkin seed course combination

Lunch:
Left-over Garlic Shrimp in Coconut Milk, Tomatoes and Cilantro OR Left-over Zucchini, Pea and Spinach Pesto Risotto

Snack: Celery sticks with guacamole

Dinner:
Taco Salad or Wild Rice Burrito Bowl with Cilantro Lime Avocado Dressing

Day 8

Breakfast:
5-Minutes Flourless Chocolate Banana Zucchini Muffins OR Pumpkin Blueberry Muffins

Snack: Brown rice salad, peanut butter, and a spoonful of honey or maple syrup

Lunch;
Left-over Orange poultry and salad or Orange To-Fu

Snack: Baby tomatoes tossed with black beans and avocado

Dinner:

Blackened Steak with Mango Avocado Salsa OR Smoky Tempeh using Fresh Peach and Cherry Tomato Salsa

Day 9

Breakfast:

Blueberry Pistachio Apple Sandwiches

Snack: 5-Minutes Flourless Chocolate Banana Zucchini Muffins

Lunch
Left-over Grilled Salmon with Mango Salsa or Smoky Tempeh

Snack: Corn Thins along with Guacamole

Dinner:

Jalapeno Turkey Burgers OR Spicy Vegan Portobello Mushroom Burgers

Day 10

Breakfast:
Morning Meal Egg Muffins OR Crust not as Sun-Dried Tomato Quiche

Snack: Baked sweet potato with peanut butter, banana, and cinnamon

Lunch
Cauliflower Mush Room Bowls

Snack: Roasted Chickpeas and berries

Dinner:

Left-over Cauliflower Mushroom Bowl using Jalapeno Turkey Burgers or Spicy Vegan Portobello Mushroom Burger

Day 11

Breakfast:
Blueberry Pistachio Apple Sandwiches

Snack: Raspberries and pistachios

Lunch
Avocado Chicken Waldorf SaladOR Vegan Waldorf Salad

Snack: Left-over cherry egg yolks or vegan egg yolks

Dinner:
Sweet Potato Noodles with Almond Dijon Vinaigrette

Day 12

Breakfast:

Left-over Breakfast egg yolks or vegan egg yolks

Snack: Banana pieces with vanilla butter and dusted with cocoa powder Lunch: Leftover sweet potato noodles

Lunch: Baby carrots and hummus

Dinner: Shrimp and Asparagus Sir FryOR Sweet and Sour Tofu

Day 13

Breakfast:

Sweet Potato Toast

Snack: 1 Larabar

Lunch: Avocado and shrimp salad (utilizing leftover beans)or sweet-sour and sweet tofu

Snack: Skinny Pop popcorn along with Hardboiled egg or couple of roasted Chickpeas

Dinner: Roasted Garlic and Herb Cod OR Easy Roasted Veggie Pizza Bites

Day 14

Breakfast:

Sweet Potato Toast

Snack: Cucumber pieces and hummus

Lunch: Leftover roasted herb and garlic codSnack: Larabar

Dinner:

Sheet Pan Chili Lime Shrimp Fajitas OR One-pan Mexican Quinoa

Day 15

Breakfast:

Berries, Beef and Coconut Shreds Cereal

Snack: Dried, pitted dates along with Peanut-butter

Lunch: Citrus Chicken Strips over Spinach Salad

Snack: Hard Boiled eggs or couple roasted chickpeas and carrots with hummus

Dinner: Tomato Basil Soup

Day 16

Breakfast:
Apple Spice Overnight Oats

Snack: Brown rice with peanut butter and banana pieces

Lunch: Left-over tomato noodle soup

Snack: Raw pepper strips together with hummus and pumpkin

Dinner:

Harvest Chicken Salad OR Lentil Cucumber Salad

Day 17

Breakfast:

Left-over: Apple Spice Overnight Oats

Snack: Dried bread and dates

Lunch:
Left-over Harvest chicken salad OR lentil cucumber salad

Snack: Apple and couple roasted chickpeas

Dinner: Steak and Veggie Quinoa Casserole OR Vegan Shepard's Pie with Gravy

Day 18

Breakfast:
Fresh fruit and Rice Breakfast Pudding

Snack: Banana and pistachios

Lunch:
Greek Quinoa Salad

Snack: Chocolate Cherry Energy Bites

Dinner: Left Overs: Chicken and Veggie Quinoa Casserole

Day 19

Breakfast:

Black Bean Scramble OR Spiced Chickpea Breakfast Scramble

Snack: Chocolate Cherry Energy Bites

Lunch:

Left Overs: Green Quinoa Salad

Snack: 100 percent apple chips and walnuts

Dinner:

Home-made Chicken Noodle Soup or Curried Lentil Butternut Squash Soup

Day 20

Breakfast:
Banana Oat Protein Muffins

Snack: Apple chips dipped in peanut butter

Lunch:
Left-over Homemade Chicken Noodle Soup or Curried Butternut Squash Soup

Snack: Chocolate Cherry Energy Bites

Dinner: Steak Fajita Nachos(I propose having"Mary's Gone Crackers" rather than creating homemade bread):

Day 21

Breakfast:
Left-over Banana oat protein muffins Snack: Chewy Lemon Oatmeal Bites

Lunch: Cashew Tuna Salad Cucumber Bites(utilize a vegan mayo) OR Simple Chickpea Salad with Tomato

Snack: Baby tomatoes and pineapple pieces tossed in olive oil, balsamic vinegar plus a pinch of pepper

Dinner:

Create Ahead Grilled Chicken and Veggie Bowls(makes 8 servings to get for your week) or Chick-pea Taco BuddhaBowl

5 TRUTH PRACTICALLY EVERYBODY MAKES SIRTFOOD DIET

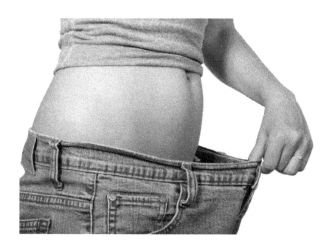

1. Eating Foods That You Can Not Actually Like

In case You believe you are going to turn into a fan of Brussels sprouts as it's January second and you've not eaten anything in the previous 3 months weeks, you are setting yourself up to fail. "One explanation diets do not work is they induce people to eat things that they don't really like. "If the carrot smoothie isn't exercising for you, take to sautéed lettuce, celery, tofu chips, or even better, ditch the carrot and attempt lettuce, collard greens, Swiss chard, or still another vegetable" The following secret to eating healthy without quitting life would be really to test out spices. "Do not forget to take to various seasonings or manners of cooking. By way of instance, get a Cajun spice combination or five-spice and scatter it together with one's poultry or veggies.

2. Expecting Immediate Results

The Observing you did on Christmas isn't going to become reversed following weekly --or possibly per couple to having the sh*t together (i.e., healthy eating). "The most straightforward way to fall short of one's resolution or goal is to help it become unattainable., lead nourishment specialist at Seattle Sutton's Healthy Eating. "For example, resolving to prevent eat your favorite take out food or planning to lose 10 lbs within 1 month may backfire. That is not because allowing the foods that you like results in finally bingeing to them once you can not tolerate the craving . And seeking to reduce a lot of weight too fast will undoubtedly cause disappointment and also a dip bag of Dorritos.

The Key would be to put smaller goals that buildup to an objective, he states. This means that you may attempt to prevent this take out joint more frequently than you can today or wish to lose a couple of pounds weekly --and soon you finally reach your target, " she states.

3. Maybe not Getting Meals in Front of Time

One of the reasons why people overeat around Christmas is there is a large amount of food outside; it is easy to catch. Whenever the observing is finished, make it simple to choose healthful options by organizing healthy food beforehand. Like that, it is possible to arrive at it when you are hungry, rather than earning a game-time decision when you are mesmerized. "Meal preparation is critical to eating a balanced diet program. "Cut vegetables up and also make additional portions of dinner to the week beforehand. In this manner, it is possible to very quickly collect dinner to a busy week."

Now you won't think some of the strangest things a few individuals did to eliminate weight:

4. Maybe not Assessing Labels at the Supermarket

Being A little more particular regarding the foods that you buy at the store will be able to assist you in getting right back on the right track after ingestion that which without any difficulty. Examine the food labels to the ingredients you have to produce a more informed decision regarding whether it belongs in what you eat plan. Chen says it especially crucial to pay careful attention to serving sizes. "A jar of juice might actually comprise two portions," she states. This means it includes twice the calories and sugar just as what's recorded on the tag. And as you are not likely in the habit of just drinking half a juice, then which will prevent you from losing weight," says Chen. Other critical elements to consider will be the total amount of protein and fiber in meals. Take 2 g of fiber and 20 g of protein into every meal to remain full and fulfilled.

5. Maybe not Acquiring a Backup Policy for Seconds Weakness

Putting A strategy set up to modify your daily diet is fantastic. However, you've also must policy for roadblocks. Simply take stress eating throughout an especially annoying afternoon, such as. Once you learn, you are enticed to make your self feel a lot better with the assistance of ice cream, then look for a backup program. Maybe you opt to find yourself a 20-minute massage at a nail salon or blow some steam off from the particular candlelight yoga class. "Both are welcome adjustments to a healthier new way of life, and you'll feel far better in the long term."

SUMMARY

Sirtfood Diet program is an idea it is possible to embark on, but perhaps not merely for weight loss but also for several due procedures indoors and out human body posture.

The Plan asserts that eating particular foods can trigger your "lean receptor" pathway and possess you losing seven pounds in 7 days. Foods such as ginseng, dark chocolate, and milk contain a natural compound called polyphenols, which mimic the results of fasting and exercise. Strawberries, red onions, cinnamon, and garlic will also be powerful sirtfoods. These foods can activate the sirtuin pathway to help activate weight reduction. The science seems appealing; however, the truth is there is very little research to back up these claims. Plus, the guaranteed speed of weight reduction from the very first week is quite quick and perhaps not in accord with the National Institute of Health's safe fat loss recommendations of a couple of pounds each week.

The Diet contains two stages:

Phase 1 lasts for 7 days. For the initial 3 days, you only drink three sirtfood green juices along with something meal full of sirtfoods for an overall total of 1000 calories. On days four through seven, you drink 2 green juices along with 2 meals for a total of 1,500 calories.

Phase Two is really a 14day maintenance program, though it's created to your shed weight steadily (perhaps not sustain your present weight). Daily is composed of three balanced sirtfood meals plus also one green juice.

Later Those 3 weeks, you are invited to keep on eating a diet full of Sirtfoods and drinking a green juice each day. You can Discover several sirtfood Cookbooks recipes and online on the sirtfood site. 1 green juice recipe Entirely on the sirtfood internet site is made up of a combination of spinach and other leafy vegetables Greens, celery, carrot, green apple, ginger, lemon juice, and matcha. Buckwheat And lovage may also be things that can be advocated for use on your green juice. The diet urges that apples should be made in a juicer, Not Just a blender; therefore, It tastes better.

CPSIA information can be obtained
at www.ICGtesting.com
Printed in the USA
LVHW051726181020
669109LV00035B/1161